Developing the
New Assertive Nurse

The authors developed the educational program Assertiveness for Nurses, upon which this book is based, as a result of their interest in the women's movement and a commitment to advancing the nursing profession. Together they have generated educational programs that have been offered continuously in numerous locations and formats for a variety of health care agencies.

Gerry Angel, R.N., M.N.Ed., provides community-based continuing education programs for Registered Nurses in Pittsburgh, Pennsylvania, which has made her increasingly aware of the conflicts and dilemmas experienced by nurses. In 1977 she initiated Assertiveness for Nurses as a team project with Ms. Petronko. Her experience includes practice in psychiatric-mental health nursing and collegiate nursing education. At present she is self-employed as a continuing education provider, counselor, and consultant to individuals and agencies in the areas of nursing career development and human relations.

Diane Knox Petronko, R.N., M.P.H., is currently associated with the Visiting Nurses Association of Allegheny County, Pittsburgh, Pennsylvania, in addition to conducting independent educational programs. Since the early 1970s she has been involved with integrating feminist philosophy into the nursing profession. Her educational experience includes graduate research in organizational theory, and she has taught Assertiveness for Women at Drake University, Des Moines, Iowa. In addition, she has wide clinical and administrative experience in community health nursing.

Developing the
New Assertive Nurse

Essentials for Advancement

GERRY ANGEL, R.N., M.N.Ed.
DIANE KNOX PETRONKO, R.N., M.P.H.

Springer Publishing Company
New York

To a New Era of Assertive Nurses.

G. A.

To Denny.

D. K. P.

Springer Publishing Company, Inc.
200 Park Avenue South
New York, New York 10003

83 84 85 86 87 / 10 9 8 7 6 5 4 3 2 1

Library of Congress Cataloging in Publication Data

Angel, Gerry.
  Developing the new assertive nurse.
  Includes bibliographies and index.
  1. Nurses—Psychology. 2. Assertiveness (Psychology) I. Petronko, Diane Knox. II. Title. [DNLM: 1. Assertiveness. 2. Nurses—Psychology. WY 87 A581d]
RT86.A53   1983   610.83'01'9   83-608
ISBN 0-8261-3511-0 (pbk.)

Printed in the United States of America

Contents

Preface

This book is an outgrowth of the authors' extensive experience in conducting assertiveness courses and workshops for hundreds of nurses functioning in a variety of clinical, administrative, and educational positions in health care agencies.

It is written for all nurses interested in growing both personally and professionally, especially those who are committed to the further development of the nursing profession. It will not only orient nurses who are unfamiliar with the principles of assertiveness but can also serve as reinforcement and expansion for those with previous exposure to courses or workshops on the topic. Even those nurses who consider themselves to be assertive can benefit from this book by gaining insight into the dilemmas their colleagues face and by learning the benefits of collegial support since the majority of examples presented are based on authentic situations from our course/workshop participants. Nurses who acquire assertiveness skills can, in turn, help patients function assertively and assume more responsibility for their own health care.

The purpose of the book is to share the concepts of assertiveness within a practical framework so that those nurses *who choose* can learn to function assertively. While we believe that assertiveness is imperative for our profession to advance, it need not be utilized by all nurses all of the time in all situations. Implementation of assertive skills depends on an individual's willingness and readiness to use them as well as on their appropriateness in a given situation. We believe that it is important to help nurses become increasingly more aware of their own feelings and values, and to identify how these variables affect behavior, particularly the individual nurse's decision regarding the situations in which she chooses to be assertive. Throughout the text, we encourage nurses to evaluate the advantages and disadvantages of assertive behavior and to decide for themselves when to function assertively. We hope that the concepts presented in the following pages reflect a true spirit of "freedom of choice."

The principles of assertiveness are applicable to both men and women, as the participation of both male and female nurses in our educational programs has revealed. However, many sections of the book address problems and concerns resulting from the fact that the nursing profession is comprised primarily of women.

Although assertiveness can be effective, it is not a "cure-all" for pronounced individual or organizational conflicts, or for all the dilemmas of the nursing profession. Often nurses must be helped to deal with underlying issues and encouraged to devote sufficient time to planning and decision making rather than focusing exclusively on the presenting problem. Both the planning and decision-making processes are necessary prerequisites to responsible assertive behavior.

Internalization of assertiveness concepts can help nurses to increase self-esteem and gain more self-control. It is important for nurses to assume more control and responsibility for their own personal and professional lives rather than allowing themselves to be victims of situations and systems. This concept of self-control is crucial. Additionally, we are convinced of the value and uniqueness of each individual and believe that in human relationships all individuals have personal rights worthy of consideration. Consequently, our approach to assertiveness emphasizes the empathic component, indicating understanding and respect for the other person.

The book progresses from specific to broad application of assertiveness concepts. Because any group is only as effective as its individual members, the major portions of the book are focused on helping the individual nurse acquire assertive skills in personal and professional aspects of her life. However, in order for assertiveness to have a positive impact on patient care and contribute to the advancement of nurses and nursing, it must be supported and developed by nursing educators and nursing managers. Consequently, the text concludes with a discussion of these issues and presents ways in which assertiveness can be used as an effective means of implementing change.

Our intent is not to substitute the book for an experiential course or workshop but rather to encourage its use in a supplemental manner. By receiving guidance from a qualified group leader, obtaining feedback and support from group members, trying out the assertive skills, and hearing how others handle their situations, the learner has a greater opportunity to internalize the assertive concepts and to change behavior than if she proceeded alone, without the advantages of a group experience.

Because the development of lasting behavioral change requires time, assertive concepts should, ideally, be taught over a period of weeks in course form, with planned follow-up sessions. The concepts can be taught as continuing education and staff development offerings. Enduring effects can also be promoted by presenting and reinforcing the concepts throughout a student's basic nursing educational program. Hopefully, nurses reading this book will be stimulated to provide for the availability of ongoing educational programs on assertiveness for nurses in their respective locations.

Acknowledgments

We wish to acknowledge our adaptation of the following informational sources: *The New Assertive Woman* by Lynn Bloom, Karen Coburn, and Joan Pearlman; the content and experience acquired from Anne Schodde and Marie Wilson through the Division of Women's Programs at Drake University.

We also want to recognize all of our course/workshop participants who have provided us with countless hours of experience and whose authentic situations have supplied the basis of many of the examples mentioned throughout the book. We are grateful to the numerous sponsors of our educational programs on Assertiveness for Nurses, especially those who initially took a risk in offering such a program, long before the topic was written about or accepted by the nursing community.

Our husbands, parents, children, colleagues, friends, and editor/typist all had a positive influence on the writing of this book. For their many contributions, we are grateful.

Gerry Angel
Diane Knox Petronko

A Special Note

During the writing of this book, we were perplexed periodically by the pronoun problem, or more specifically, the "he/she" issue. We recognize the importance of expressing the equality of the sexes. However, we believe that a "himself/herself" in the middle of a sentence often reduces its impact.

Consequently, we have chosen to deal with the dilemma in this manner: Since currently 96.4 percent of the nursing profession is female, pronouns referring to "the nurse" in the book are written in the feminine gender. This is not to neglect the male members of the profession but simply to make the grammatical pronoun usage less cumbersome. On the other hand, when we make general references to individuals outside the nursing profession, the masculine pronoun is used. After much deliberation, we determined that this solution represents an acceptable compromise while maintaining a forceful writing style.

The Importance of Assertiveness for Nurses

As children, we are generally open, honest, and outspoken, sometimes to the embarrassment of adults. By the time we become adults, we behave differently because we have been socialized according to the expectations of our environment. This socialization process makes it possible for large numbers of people to coexist with a minimum amount of daily conflict in a complex world. However, some portions of the socialization process may have influenced us to such an extent that we are restricted by them. To recapture some of the attributes of our childhood, we need to open ourselves to the processes of reevaluation and reeducation of our attitudes and behavior.

Why Aren't Nurses Naturally Assertive?

To answer the question of why nurses are not naturally assertive, one needs first to acknowledge that 96.4 percent of all nurses in the United States are women, who have experienced socialization via society's expectations of females. From birth, boys and girls are treated differently and, consequently, internalize different standards for "acceptable" behavior. A little boy is seldom discouraged from being "rough," boisterous, or competitive in the way a little girl is; a young girl frequently is given messages to stay neat and clean, to be reserved, and to "know her place." In later years, similar behavior exhibited by adult men and women is perceived differently by society. For instance, when a man actively pursues a goal, he is seen as "successful"; a woman acting in the same manner is viewed as "pushy." Health care team members generally accept a male physician who throws a temper tantrum when his favorite equipment is unavailable for a procedure; a similar aggressive outburst from a female nursing supervisor would be considered childish and unprofessional. In general, women are rewarded for being "nice," "passive," and "receptive." The "perfect little woman" is still seen as the good listener, who is a little shy in public and consistently places her family and friends' needs before her own.

Young women receive these messages very early. When a young woman announces that she wants to become a nurse, responses can convey one of two messages that are based on the stereotype of the self-sacrificing, submissive nurse. The seemingly positive reaction may be "Marvelous, nursing is a good field for a woman. It prepares you for marriage and motherhood and is something you can always fall back on." The second, seemingly more negative, response may be "Why be a nurse? If you insist on higher education, you should choose something more challenging like medicine, engineering, or law." In this second case, the message is that anyone can be a nurse. The result of such stereotyping is that nurses often have a conflicting image—that of a devoted but not respected caregiver. To gain more insight into this matter, it is helpful to consider some relevant aspects of the history of nursing and nursing education in the United States.

In the late 1800s the primary setting for nursing education was the hospital, a place for the poor and homeless to receive care. While the cause was noble, association with such a deplorable setting was not prestigious. Within these substandard facilities, nurses' duties were scarcely distinguishable from those of a servant. Nurses cleaned, cooked, laundered clothes, and tended fires. They bathed and fed the patients and carried out physicians' orders. One must ask whether these nurses were students or laborers (Ashley, 1976).

These early hospital schools of nursing in the United States were influenced by Florence Nightingale's system of nursing education. However, Nightingale's approach was modified in the United States, where schools did not have independent administration and financing, and were controlled by hospitals and physicians. From the very beginning of formalized nursing education, the practice of nursing was not autonomous; rather, it was dependent on male-dominated institutions.

Nurses were trained by the apprenticeship system, which can be viewed as an optimum way of keeping a female group in subjection to a male-dominated group (Ashley, 1976). Male physicians provided what little formal nursing education existed, and they determined what nurses needed to know and when.

Early nursing educators encouraged humility and fostered low self-esteem in their students. Physicians, who did not agree with improving the quality of nursing education, went so far as to stress that nurses should never try to be seen as learned or valuable (Ashley, 1976). With such a history, it is not surprising that nurses as a group have low self-esteem!

During the early 1900s American women were "put on a pedestal" and told that they were special; yet they were denied the right to vote. In parallel with women in general, nurses were given a similar double message. On one hand, nurses were told that they had a special calling: Their devotion and dedication truly made them "angels of mercy" and, thus, ideal women. They were told that the hospital could not run without them. On the other hand, they were treated as inferior workers, subservient to physicians, and were kept oppressed and powerless. Some writers (Ehrenreich and English, 1973a) believe that the repression of female health care workers was part of a sex and class struggle, and that the newly developing medical profession usurped the role of women healers, allowing the nursing profession to continue because nurses were viewed as harmless and helpful.

Nurses had no power or claim to the credit of healing, for they were expected to utilize all the womanly traits of caring, nurturing, and soothing while leaving the gathering of data, analyzing, decision making, and recommending to the male physician and paternalistic hospital administration. Nurses were given the message not to be concerned with matters of reasonable hours, fair wages, and decent working conditions. Indeed, they were taught that speaking out violated not only their "professionalism" but their very femininity (Ehrenreich and English, 1973b). Mauksch (1980) believes that this issue helps to clarify why nursing and medicine took separate paths. Nurses were submissive and did not speak out about their wages or their working conditions, even in the interest of patients. They just kept quiet and "made do," whereas physicians were outspoken and demanding about the resources and equipment they needed to provide medical care. This important difference may help to explain how the roles of autonomous physician and subservient nurse developed.

These attitudes did not change much during the mid-1900s. Although the quality of nursing education improved somewhat and a movement began to locate schools of nursing in an academic setting, the majority of nurses continued to be prepared in hospital diploma schools of nursing. While other health care professions quickly established their educational preparation in academia, nursing education remained predominantly outside the mainstream of professional education. For a long time, the priority in diploma schools was to provide nursing service for the hospital rather than to educate students. Students were expected to please the authority figures and to conform. Assertive students were systematically stifled or asked to leave.

The passive, second-class orientation stressed in nursing schools and fostered in practice settings continued after graduation into the work world. The paternalistic hospital system thrived in the early 1900s when most nurses lived on the hospital grounds. Nurses worked 12-hour days, often with split shifts, for meager wages; but they were "taken care of"—that is, the hospital provided free room and board. Is it any wonder that soon after marriage most nurses left? Along this line, it is important to remember that nursing was considered excellent training for marriage. Understandably, most nurses, identifying themselves as "only nurses," were not career oriented and did not view themselves as professionals with accompanying esteem, rights, and privileges. Because many nurses left the work force to raise a family, they had little intention of maintaining a continuous, lifelong career, and so few made a professional commitment to devote themselves to advancing the nursing profession.

These aborted and interrupted work careers, combined with the philosophy of nursing education at the time and the way nurses were treated (and permitted themselves to be treated) in the systems in which they worked, contributed to a serious lack of professional advancement. Nurses did not have the confidence to assert themselves, to speak out on an issue, or to ask for what they wanted; nor were they given the encouragement or support to do so. Fortunately, this orientation was to be affected by future events.

Why Learn Principles of Assertiveness?

The interest of individual nurses in learning to be assertive is a natural outgrowth of the economic, social, and professional developments of the 1970s.

Indirectly, economic factors have influenced nurses to desire more assertive behavior. The two-paycheck family has become a necessity, and nurses have finally decided that if they are going to work, it is not beneath their "dignity" to be concerned with wages, benefits, and job security. The increased involvement of nurses in collective bargaining clearly supports that notion.

Although organized nursing was not in the vanguard of the women's movement, the profession has benefited from the movement's gains and influence. When the women's movement addressed the problems of women in the workplace, nurses began to consider the potential safety hazards of air-polluted operating rooms and other work settings and to evaluate their salaries and benefits in relation to comparable male positions. The ideas of regarding nursing as something merely "to fall back on" and working for "pin money" began to fade as nurses joined with other women to affirm their right to pursue a career seriously. The feminist movement helped mothers who worked outside the home to become more socially acceptable. Likewise, nursing leaders made significant gains in upgrading the educational preparation of nurses and in fostering a stronger professional commitment toward advancement of the profession. Nurses began to recognize that it was permissible to work because they enjoyed nursing and that such a career could be self-actualizing.

The feminist movement has had a major impact on nursing in that it has helped the profession to recognize that many of its problems are related to its predominantly female composition. Nurses collectively are treated by the health care industry as one composite woman. This new perspective has enhanced a greater understanding of the factors that influenced the development of the profession and of the steps necessary to change the direction of nursing from subservience to autonomy. These new outlooks have created an environment in which nurses have begun to assess their individual needs.

The 1970s have been called the decade of the "me generation" because during that period many Americans, enjoying comfortable life-styles, became introspective and more demanding of self-actualizing leisure and work activities. During this decade, women especially evaluated their personal developmental needs and began planning to meet them. Such a movement was also present within the nursing profession, as evidenced by the writings of Kramer (1974). New graduates were not as passive as their predecessors; they came to their first jobs with expectations, and when they became frustrated, they often left. As established nurses explored their professional identities within complex health care delivery systems, they began questioning what personal rewards they were reaping. This search led many nurses to take a fresh look at their often receptive, "victim" behaviors (Dean, 1978), and many decided that they wanted a new professional stance.

Much writing and research was prompted as nurses began exploring the identity issue. Reports revealed a low self-esteem among nurses and identified contributing factors. For example, history certainly indicated that from the very beginning, nursing had been defined and controlled by others. Furthermore, Greenleaf (1978) points out that it had become beneficial to the American economic system for nurses to feel inferior because if nurses valued their work highly, they would expect higher salaries. Ashley (1976) and Heide (1973) point out that nurses and women as a group have experienced similar oppressive factors which contributed to their low self-esteem: Neither group has performed work that was valued by society, and neither group has had access to power. Greenleaf (1978) suggests that one initial way for nurses to establish power is to develop self-confidence in their competency. Consequently, self-esteem will evolve, and from this a power base can be established. Indeed, nurses have begun to speak, write, and concern themselves with rights and power.

As might be expected of a newly awakened oppressed group,

nurses no longer want to be victims of male-dominated health care systems, and they are beginning to demand control over their personal and professional lives. Once the initial anger and indignation subsided, nurses were faced with the real challenge of implementing changes they had identified as necessary for nursing to become a fully developed, autonomous, and accountable health profession. In accepting this opportunity to set new directions for the profession, the development of assertive skills can help nurses to chart a new course.

In addition to movements from outside the profession, certain other relevant happenings occurred within the nursing profession itself. One such change was that nurses found that they were expected to accept and internalize significant departures from traditional nursing theory and practice. As new technologies developed, nurses assumed more specialized, complex responsibility for patient care and often found the accompanying accountability frightening. Additionally, nurses were expected to acquire advanced educational preparation, to function more autonomously, to make nursing diagnoses, and to initiate, implement, and evaluate a plan of care. After years of subordination to physicians, nurses were expected to confer with them as colleagues, a position which was difficult to achieve. It was soon apparent that nurses needed more than knowledge and technical skills: They also needed to believe in themselves.

These simultaneously increasing demands from society and the nursing profession led to turmoil, both individual and intraprofessional. As new ideas filtered down to individual nurses, it became evident that many nurses lacked the communication and behavioral skills required to deal with this turbulence and to be effective change agents. Recently, many nurses have found that the acquisition of assertive skills is one effective way to meet the current and future challenges of their profession.

What Is Assertiveness?

Assertiveness is open, honest, and direct communication that takes into consideration your own personal rights as well as the rights of others. "Integrity" is a key concept in that one's own in-

tegrity and the integrity of others are preserved and enhanced.
Simply stated, assertiveness is saying no when you really want to
say no and saying yes when you really want to say yes. It is a way
of increasing your self-confidence and of saying what you feel without undermining others, thereby allowing you to gain more self-
respect as well as respect from others. Assertiveness is also a way
to stop being a victim of situations and systems; instead, assertiveness allows you to recognize and explore the alternatives in a
given situation and to initiate their implementation if you so desire.

The goals of assertiveness are twofold:

1. To stand up for your personal rights without infringing on
   the rights of others
2. To reduce anxiety which often prevents us from behaving
   assertively and (a) locks us into passive behavior where
   our own rights are denied or (b) precipitates an aggressive
   outburst where the rights of others are violated

Assertiveness is not a method to gain control over others or
to "beat the system" but rather is a way of dealing with others in a
self-satisfying and respectful way. Through assertiveness, you
may not always get what you want, but hopefully you will feel better about yourself. Assertiveness can help you to make choices and
to determine who you are and who you want to be. Learning assertiveness principles and techniques can help you develop the skills
and strength to be your own person. Once individuals learn to be
assertive, they have a skill that allows them more choices, more independence, and more control over their own lives (Bloom, Coburn,
and Pearlman, 1975).

How Assertiveness Differs from Passive
and Aggressive Behavior

Assertive behavior differs from both passive behavior and aggressive behavior. The following contrast is based on the writing
of Bloom, Coburn, and Pearlman (1975). Characteristically, the

passive person is acted upon by being the recipient or object of action. Passivity is often self-denying and often carries with it some subtle hostility. The passive person seeks to avoid responsibility and is typically the victim or martyr. Although the intent of passive behavior is to avoid conflict and confrontation, in reality, these are often provoked.

The aggressive person, on the other hand, is usually the "attacker" and is active in initiating movements in an offensive way. Aggressive behavior is selfish behavior. Its intent is to put down, to dominate, and to win at another's expense. Aggressive people often speak in "you" statements that place blame or undue responsibility on the other person.

In contrast to both passive and aggressive behavior, assertiveness involves putting oneself forward by way of a positive declaration. The intent of assertive behavior is to express and to communicate in an atmosphere of trust and mutual concern. Characteristically, assertiveness is self-fulfilling, self-enhancing, and self-actualizing. Assertive people speak in "I" statements that take responsibility and attempt to offer a solution.

Each of these behavior types can take a variety of forms. The examples that follow illustrate some of these forms.

Situation 1

Mr. Jones, a patient on your unit, is allergic to penicillin. There is a notice on the front of his chart indicating this fact. After reviewing the results of his culture and sensitivity, the physician decides that an antibiotic is needed and proceeds to order penicillin. As the nurse, you might respond in a variety of ways:

Passive Response

1. Out of fear of contradicting the physician, you remain silent and let the order stand, hoping that someone else will take responsibility for correcting it.

2. You say nothing directly to the physician, but you quickly tell the head nurse and let her deal with the situation.

3. In a barely audible, hesitant manner, with little eye contact, you stammer, "Doctor, uhh . . . do you know . . . Mr. Jones is . . . uhh . . . allergic to penicillin?"

Aggressive Response

1. Standing with hands on hips and conveying an attitude of superiority, you say, "Are you out of your mind? You know Mr. Jones is allergic to penicillin!"
2. Sarcastically, you ask, "What medical school did you graduate from? Ordering penicillin for a patient who's allergic to it—you would think you'd know better!"

Assertive Response

1. You state the facts in a nonjudgmental way: "Mr. Jones is allergic to penicillin. What else would you like to order?"

Situation 2

You and an aide are working the 3:00-to-11:00 P.M. shift, and you are hurriedly trying to complete your charting. Three lights go on from patients' rooms, and you see the aide walking down the hall with her coat, ready to leave.

Passive Response

1. You say nothing but feel hurt or angry inside that you are being left with all the work.
2. You take a deep breath, sigh, and say softly to yourself in a resigned manner, "I guess I'll be here until midnight." As you watch the aide make her exit, you feel like a martyr as well as a victim of circumstances.
3. It takes all you have, but you muster up enough courage to say hesitatingly and pleadingly, "Uhh, Mary . . . do you

think ... you could come back ... and ... give me a hand ... huh?"

Aggressive Response

1. You get up from your charting and yell down the hall in a derogatory and commanding way, "Mary, where do you think you're going? Get back here and answer these lights!"

2. After calling Mary back to the office, you proceed to belittle her and condemn her by saying, "Mary, what's wrong with you? Don't you know better than to walk out early on a busy night? Your sense of responsibility leaves a lot to be desired."

Assertive Response

1. In a firm, assured, manner, you call the aide back to the nurses' station and say to her, "Mary, I know you're in a hurry to leave, but there are ten minutes left before the shift is over. I've got a lot of charting to do. If you help by answering the patients' lights and I work on the charts, hopefully we'll both be able to leave at a reasonable hour."

Discussion of Situations

Hopefully, these brief examples help to clarify what assertiveness is and what it is not. A common misconception is that assertiveness equates with oppressive behavior. Once individuals understand assertiveness and how it differs from aggression, they are much more receptive to the concept. The following comment made by a nursing manager bears this out: "When my staff returned from Assertiveness for Nurses, I expected an aggressive barrage of dissatisfaction with our system. What I got were staff members who communicate openly, directly, and effectively about the things that really count in this organization."

Many nursing administrators, managers, and educators who refine their own assertive skills recognize the benefits of supporting and developing assertive staff, faculty, and students. They realize that assertive nurses do not avoid the conflict that is inherent in complex organizations but instead manage it and make decisions. Furthermore, assertive nurses view all members of the health care team as colleagues and have equal relationships with physicians and other co-workers.

Assertive nurses are also satisfied with themselves and their work performance. Consequently, they are more likely to remain in a given setting for a period of time, thereby contributing to the reduction of staff turnover. Importantly, assertive nurses set appropriate limits and do not jeopardize safe patient care, good management, or sound educational principles by assuming excessive responsibility. They are goal oriented and initiate ideas rather than merely reacting to the ideas of others. Assertive nurses are an asset to an organization because they can be counted on to communicate directly and effectively without "playing games" or being devious and manipulative. *Tell What U Want.*

Such open, honest, and direct communication, however, does not occur frequently enough. Instead, many individuals engage in interpersonal, nonassertive "games" as a way of coping with life's situations.   *11/13/01*
                                                                                         Bodell

Game Playing: A Nonassertive Way of Communicating

Although the "games" considered in this section have relevance to Berne's *Games People Play* (1964), the following discussion of the games nurses play, within the context of the health care system, is based upon material presented by Bloom, Coburn, and Pearlman (1975). Unlike Berne, these authors use the term "game" to refer to an indirect, manipulative form of nonassertive behavior by which the player tries to get what is desired in a subversive way, without asking for it.

Unfortunately, our society promotes hypocrisy and discourages openness and truthfulness in the name of tact or consideration (Lazarus, 1974). As a result, the games we have been taught to play are really exercises in nonassertive behavior. They have become so ingrained in our functioning that many times we are unaware of even playing them. They are used at one time or another by all of us and, if carried to extremes, can become pathological. For purposes of this book, however, the discussion of "games people play" is confined to "normal" usage.

The use of games evolves primarily out of fear of the eventual outcome of a situation and is an attempt to escape anxiety and antagonism. An individual's strong desire to have needs met while still feeling liked and accepted by others provides additional impetus to participation in manipulative game playing.

The following sections offer descriptions of specific types of games, offering you the opportunity to do some introspection and examination of the extent to which you participate in any or all of them. Recognition of how you currently function is a vital prerequisite to becoming assertive.

The "Suffering" Game

The "sufferer," or martyr, is the person who sets herself up to be overloaded or takes on tasks that are not duly hers. By conveying how taxed and overworked she is, her hope is that others will offer assistance without her requesting it directly. She presents an external facade of doing a remarkable quantity of work, while underneath she resents it and gripes about it. Her pattern is to take on more than she can handle comfortably, even to the extent of sometimes performing tasks that others refuse to do and subordinating her own work to theirs. Although not conveyed directly, her expectation is that others will reciprocate in a like manner.

This tactic often backfires when others take advantage of the sufferer's behavior by supplying her with even more tasks. She ends up feeling as though she is existing almost solely to benefit others. This game can also backfire if others withdraw from it after recognizing that they are being manipulated into providing aid to the sufferer. Illustrations of this game can be found in numerous nursing settings.

Example 1

A front-line nursing manager wants to prove to others (as well as to herself) that she is a "supernurse." She not only performs her management responsibilities but also assumes an excessive direct patient care assignment by picking up the slack of a less competent staff member. She feels overextended and angry with her subordinate's lack of ability but tries to convince herself that she is working hard in the interest of patient care. Besides, she thinks the staff will like her because she "pitches in" and, in turn, hopes that they will help her out when her load becomes too demanding.

Example 2

As an undergraduate nursing instructor, Ann assigns all kinds of extensive requirements and clinical responsibilities to her students. She conveys to her co-workers how much her students are learning, while simultaneously complaining about how overworked she is, with numerous commitments and grades to compile. Underneath, she feels overwhelmed and hopes that the department chairperson will recognize her plight by assigning some of her students to another instructor or that one of her co-workers will help her out voluntarily.

Discussion of Examples

In each of these situations, the nurse set herself up to be overloaded, with the end result that she felt angry and resentful, hoping someone else would be perceptive and take the initiative to reduce her burden. The assertive alternative to "suffering" is to set limits for yourself regarding what you will and will not do, to be certain of your goals, and to state your expectations clearly while recognizing that others also have rights.

In the first example, the nursing manager could be more effective with her subordinate by helping her to sharpen her skills or to organize her work better so as to function more competently, instead of assuming patient care responsibility for her. By reevaluating the purposes of her assignments to the students, the nursing educator in the second example could reduce the quantity and improve the quality of a limited number of assignments, thus making her own job more manageable. Another option would be to ask assertively for help instead of waiting passively for someone to provide it.

The "Uninvolved" Game

The person who remains detached and "uninvolved" is hesitant to commit herself, often out of fear of antagonizing others. Typically, she never takes a stand. Consequently, she is conveniently never right or wrong. She defers to others in order to avoid responsibility, decision making, and the risk of possible accompanying conflict. Her attitude is one of apathy or noncommital acceptance of others' decisions. Denial of her true feelings is frequently accompanied by innumerable rationalizations.

While attempting to convey outward approval of another's behavior, such nonassertive dishonesty is saturated with inner resentment. Ironically, not only is the initiator of this behavior disgruntled, but often her behavior precipitates the very thing she fears: antagonism of others. People may withdraw from her out of lack of respect or become angry because of her indifference and reluctance to make a commitment.

The following illustrations give examples of the game of uninvolvement in the nursing world.

Example 1

As a staff nurse, Joan is displeased with the current method of patient care assignments on her unit. She has a new idea that she would like to see implemented but is fearful of making a suggestion because she is afraid the head nurse might interpret the ideas as a personal criticism of her ability and become antagonistic. Although this concern may be realistic, there is also the possibility of a positive outcome. To avoid a possible negative outcome, Joan completes her assignments in a routine way, feeling internal dissatisfaction and external detachment and uninvolvement from the major workings of her unit.

Example 2

Terry has been working in a given facility for a number of years as an oncology specialist and has proven herself very competent and well respected in the field. Lately, however, she had felt the need for change and would like to assume an administrative position within the same setting. Unaware of Terry's interest in administration, the director of nursing mentions to her that an assistant director position will be available soon and that she is contemplating appointing one of Terry's colleagues to the position. Even though Terry would like to be considered, she is fearful of letting her desires be known. She thinks to herself, "I may not be selected, and, if I am, I may not do the job adequately." When the director asks Terry's opinion of the nurse being considered for the position, Terry responds with, "Gee, I don't know . . . whatever you think is best. You're certainly the one to judge who can handle that position."

Discussion of Examples

In each of these examples, the nurse wanted to take the initiative—either to change a routine or to change her position. However, because she feared the possibility of evoking antagonism or of assuming the risks and responsibilities involved in making her wishes known, she remained aloof and uninvolved.

If the staff nurse had expressed her idea for a new patient care assignment routine, it may or may not have been accepted favorably, but chances are she would have felt better about herself as a result and, consequently, would not have found it necessary to play the game of uninvolvement. Similarly, if the clinical specialist had communicated openly her desire for the position in question, she may or may not have been appointed, but she probably would have felt better about herself by letting her desires be known.

One possible detrimental consequence of playing the uninvolved game is inner resentment. An individual's feelings are often disproportionately displaced onto someone or something totally removed from the underlying conflict situation.

The assertive alternative to being uninvolved is to communicate in an open, honest, and direct way and to accept the risks and responsibilities that such behavior entails. Obviously, sometimes this is easier said than done. It is not unusual for psychological impediments to prevent that from happening. (These impediments are discussed in Chapter 5.)

Certainly, there are appropriate times when one may choose not to get involved in a particular situation after examining the possible risks and consequences. For example, a particular director of nursing was having lunch with the department heads of pharmacy and medicine. When a conflict situation arose regarding the control of experimental drugs in the facility, the director of nursing decided that the problem belonged to the other departments and that it was in her best interest not to get involved. When asked for her opinion, she stated, "That sounds like something the two of you need to work out. I'm not getting in the middle of that one!"

In this instance, she still implemented the concepts of assertiveness because she was in control of her own behavior and made a knowledgeable, purposeful choice not to get involved in the discussion. This is different from being out of control and a victim of the situation or circumstances. Further, she communicated her stance in an open, honest, and direct way. This behavior is different from participation in the uninvolved game, in which an individual is dishonest with herself and others.

The "Passive Resistance" Game

People who use "passive resistance" or "passive aggressive" behavior are passive in the sense that they do not exert initiative to let others know what they want; they hope that their manipulations will supply the necessary clues. In this respect, they are similar to the sufferer described previously, but they go a step beyond by affecting others' behavior in an indirectly resistant manner. Their behavior is aggressive in that they try to accomplish their goals at all costs without regard for others. Often they criticize another's behavior without stating what they would like changed, while hoping that others will offer to be accommodating. Passive-resistive people are stubborn in wanting their own way and generally are unwilling to compromise. Dealing with them can become an either/or proposition because their attitude is typically as follows: *"Either* you guess what I want and consider it *or* I'll resist cooperating with you until you ask what I want and give it to me."* In their unwillingness to support what others want, they seek to avoid confrontation and direct conflict. "I won't fight, but I won't give you satisfaction either" is their approach.

Within the health care system, nurses and other personnel can be found playing this game. The following example helps to illustrate passive-resistant patterns of behavior.

Example

The clinical specialist in a previous example who was reluctant to apply for the administrative position easily could become passive resistant in her interactions with the newly appointed assistant director of nursing. Because she desires more authority in the setting but has not asked for it, hoping it would be supplied, her resentment probably will build. Recognizing the importance of her oncology nursing experience to the Utilization Review Committee, she could (conveniently) make herself unavailable or unnecessarily busy whenever the new assistant director, whose position she wanted, attempts to approach her about serving on the committee.

Discussion of Example

The passive-resistance game is seriously detrimental to relationships. If others do not perceive correctly what the resister wants, she may become resentful. This is especially true in close, personal relationships and is characterized by the all-too-common plea that "if you really cared about me, you'd know what I want." In extreme situations, this game can become a boggling mind-reading experiment that almost always ends in disappointment for everyone involved.

Another outcome of this game is that other people become annoyed with the resister and either ignore her or tell her off so that she ends up provoking the exact conflict she originally intended to avoid. In some cases, others may accommodate her reluctantly while harboring much resentment, ultimately losing trust in her.

The assertive alternative to such game-playing maneuvers is to foster open discussion in which understanding and mutually satisfying solutions can occur. If the clinical specialist had in the first place openly expressed her desire for the administrative position to the director of nursing, she may have had less built-up resentment, even if she had been refused the position. In addition, if she had been open and honest with herself by recognizing the effect of her lack of authority on her willingness to cooperate, she may have been able to discuss her concerns openly with the new assistant director. Although such insight and self-understanding may be difficult for some people to develop, their acquisition is invaluable.

The Game of "Sabotage"

All the games discussed thus far—suffering, uninvolvement, and passive resistance—can, in some cases, be forms of the game "sabotage." Although the saboteur does not want to comply with others' wishes, she does so in order to avoid the possibility of anger or conflict. However, she takes out her resentment in devious, manipulative, indirect ways similar to the passive resister described earlier. While the passive resister avoids complying with others' desires, the saboteur does what others want while subordinating her own desires.

Not surprisingly, the saboteur is frequently angry and frustrated. Her primary intent is to get even with those people making demands on her. Consequently, she operates with the thought "I'll do what you want, but you'll pay the price." She makes up her own set of rules, which may include such guidelines as "I'll do it my own way—when I'm good and ready—if I remember at all."

Generally, the saboteur's nonassertive behavior is contradictory and self-defeating. While she would like others to cancel their demands on her, she does not communicate that fact directly. Instead, she resorts to a series of covert tactics in an attempt to accomplish her purpose. She may procrastinate getting to the job at hand, or she may perform in an inefficient, careless way. The task may take twice as long as it should so that timetables are not met, or the job may be forgotten completely. Specifically, the saboteur may undermine the initiator of demands by spreading false rumors or organizing others to act in a retaliatory fashion.

Like the other games discussed, sabotage is played by nurses in the work setting, as the following examples illustrate.

Example 1

Although Nancy agrees to work on her day off in order to accommodate a pleading supervisor, she resents it terribly, even though she says nothing to the supervisor. In her opinion, she has been asked entirely too often to give up her scheduled time off and to rearrange personal commitments. At different times, she has considered letting the supervisor know her feelings, but she is afraid of the consequences of such a decision.

Somehow during the course of this particular unscheduled day, nothing seems to go right for Nancy. She is less efficient than usual, cannot seem to keep her mind on what she is doing, and has a number of questions, necessitating frequent calls to the supervisor who requested her to work.

Example 2

As a member of the evening i.v. team, Helen has been instructed to clean the laminar flow hood, which is a piece of equipment in which the pharmacist mixes i.v. solutions. She has been doing this job reluctantly for a number of weeks. Although she feels this is not the type of job nursing personnel should be responsible for, she is hesitant to discuss the matter with her superior for fear of retaliation. She is also afraid of instigating a conflict between the nursing and pharmacy departments since she is aware of some existing difficulties between them.

Instead, she finds herself "forgetting" to clean the laminar flow hood, or she puts the task off until the very last minute of her shift so that she may not have time to do a thorough cleaning. In fact, sometimes she even stays overtime to finish the job she forgot. Complaining constantly, she undermines the nursing administration for not having better control over nursing functions, thus exerting a destructive influence on other staff members. Generally unpleasant to be around, she has contemplated resigning but has not taken action.

Discussion of Examples

In addition to possible negative effects on others, the results of the game of sabotage are most detrimental to the saboteur herself. Her subversive behaviors (procrastination, reduced efficiency, forgetfulness, and undermining others) are all outgrowths of her frustration and suggest ineptness rather than more accurately calling attention to the excessive demands placed on her or the unreasonableness of the situation. By behaving in such a nonassertive manner and by permitting other people or circumstances to dominate her, she ends up punishing herself. Her maneuvers also may anger other people to the point that she receives the brunt of their hostility. Instead of aiding in the solution of her problems, her manipulative behavior actually intensifies them. The assertive alternative to sabotage is to discuss the problem openly and directly with the person responsible for making demands or with whomever is in a position to alter the situation.

Nancy, the staff nurse who agreed resentfully to work on her day off, could assertively discuss with the supervisor her feelings of being exploited. Also, she could say no in an assertive manner when asked to work extra. (The specifics of refusing requests assertively are discussed in Chapter 5.) Ideally, Nancy should have approached her supervisor as soon as she recognized that her willingness to cooperate was being abused. By being assertive earlier, less of her energy would have been invested in concern over the situation. Also, her chances of exploding eventually because of her inability to tolerate persistent requests would have been reduced.

Likewise, Helen could have avoided making both herself and others miserable if she had communicated in an assertive manner her dissatisfaction about cleaning pharmacy equipment. She could have conveyed her honest concern regarding the anticipated conflict between the nursing and pharmacy departments by suggesting a workable alternative and then lending her support to nursing administration.

By speaking up, both Nancy and Helen probably would have received more satisfactory results than their sabotage caused. Even if the outcomes had not been ideal, each nurse would have felt better about herself for having done what she could in a positive, constructive way.

The Game of "Seduction"

This nonassertive game is one in which women initiate flirtatious behavior in their relationships with men in order to obtain favors or privileges without asking for them directly. It is a sexual way of obtaining nonsexual goals. Such an approach is a dependent one and conveys the message that "poor little me needs big, strong, handsome you." It is based on the belief that men do not like open, honest, and direct behavior in women. The seductive nurse operates on the assumption that men are vain and egotistical, and that they consequently enjoy flattery and therefore are responsive to a female's indirect ploys.

Although traditionally men have been the "seducers" in male/ female relationships, our culture encourages women to use their femininity in a manipulative way for the purpose of getting what they want. Examples of this encouragement appear in movies, contemporary books, and television. It is not uncommon to find that the heroine in the story is a female counterspy who discovers an important plan by seducing a member of the opposition. In some writings, women are taught ways to nourish their husband's ego through manipulation and seduction in order to gain benefits for themselves (Morgan, 1973).

Most frequently, evidence of the games of seduction in health care settings can be seen between male physicians and female nurses, as the following example illustrates.

Example

Joan, the head nurse of the intensive care unit, is young and attractive. Tom, the physician in charge, is in his late 30s, is handsome, and is well respected for his medical competency. He is extremely egotistical, aggressive, and autocratic. His forceful, authoritarian demeanor causes many nurses a great deal of anxiety and discomfort. Joan soon learned that he was much more manageable when she fluttered her long eyelashes at him, grinned sheepishly, and let him know that the unit could not possibly function without him.

She makes it a point to spend time with him informally at least twice a week to seductively nurture their relationship. Although she is a very competent, skillful nurse, she never takes credit for her ability. Any major "nursing" decisions that need to be made to manage the unit are always cleared with him first. Joan takes pride in the fact that their relationship is such a "good" one, and she enjoys being the envy of her staff. She also makes it clear that unless she is completely unavailable, all communications between Tom and the nursing personnel are to be handled through her.

Discussion of Example

The results of playing the seduction game may very well be that an individual gets what she wants. In Joan's case, her patients receive good medical care. Her unit is always well supplied with equipment, medications, and sufficient personnel. Tom supports her administratively and sees that she gets whatever she needs to run an efficient unit. Because she succeeds at her goals, the game continues.

Eventually, however, the game may wear thin. Patient care can become dependent on the maintenance of a personal, seductive relationship. If something goes astray between the two individuals, patient care can be jeopardized.

This type of game playing is demeaning to both men and women because it is basically dishonest, capitalizing on the vulnerabilities of the seduced person. It may also end up being self-defeating if the seducer's indirect communication is misinterpreted. The seductress puts herself in a dependent position by being completely at the mercy of the other person to translate her message correctly.

In the example given, Tom feels free to make occasional "off-color" remarks with sexual overtones. Joan becomes embarrassed and does not know how to handle these remarks. She would prefer that they not be made at all, but she does nothing except blush because she does not want to disturb their "good" relationship. Meanwhile, not only is her own self-respect diminishing, but she is gradually losing Tom's respect as well as her staff's.

The assertive alternative to the game of seduction is direct and honest communication. If Joan relates with Tom in a straightforward manner, she may not always get what she wants. In the long run, however, she probably will gain more respect—from him, her nursing colleagues, and herself.

Summary

By participating in any or all of the games described, one may acquire short-term benefits, but the long-term results are destined to be costly. The game player gradually relinquishes her power to control her own communications by becoming increasingly dependent on others to pick up her hints and correctly interpret her covert messages. The amount of energy she spends maneuvering for short-term gains in order to escape conflict and responsibility is enormous. Eventually, the old problems resurface and may be even more severe. Games create barriers that are not easily removed.

An assertive approach makes games unnecessary. By using assertive behavior, nurses can develop their own natural resources to give them power and control while developing self-esteem, which many authors claim is lacking within the profession (Ashley, 1976; Greenleaf, 1978; Grissum and Spengler, 1976). If they desire, nurses can learn to pursue what they want directly, without waiting to see if manipulative ploys pay off.

When You Want to Be Assertive, What Do You Say?

Many nurses want to be assertive, but for a variety of reasons, some of which are mentioned at the beginning of this chapter, they do not know how. In our courses and workshops, we have found that presentation of the "Components of the Assertive Response/Approach" (Bloom, Coburn, and Pearlman, 1975), which can be used as a model for saying assertive words, is beneficial for nurses who need a specific guide to follow.

Assertive techniques are most effective when some fore-thought is given to their appropriateness in a given situation. A number of factors should be considered in advance of using these components to help you decide whether you want to be assertive. (These considerations are discussed in Chapter 2.) It is important to remember that the components should not be used in isolation but in conjunction with proper planning and decision-making skills (Chapter 6) as well as with effective communication techniques (Chapter 4).

As subsequent chapters illustrate, simply voicing assertive words may not be sufficient. In most cases, the manner in which they are said and the preparation done in advance significantly enhance the results. Individuals should say what is comfortable and "right" for them in an assertive manner. However, for those who need specific suggestions, as most of the nurses in our groups have, the following guidelines (adaptations of the work done by Bloom, Coburn, and Pearlman, 1975) should prove helpful. The components of the assertive response/approach are as follows:

EMPATHIC COMPONENT	"I understand"/I hear you" (indicates empathy)
DESCRIPTION OF FEELINGS OR SITUATION	"I feel"/"The situation is" (relates observation)
EXPECTATIONS	"I want"/"The situation requires" (conveys request)
CONSEQUENCES (POSITIVE OR NEGATIVE)	"If you do"/"If you don't" (states alternative)

The first component is the empathic one, which is not necessary in all situations. When appropriate, it enables a nurse to utilize the approach of "tuning in" to the feelings and circumstances of the other person. Most participants in our sessions adapt readily to this component because empathy traditionally has been a part of nurses' roles.

The second component consists of stating your feelings or describing the situation, whichever you prefer. It is designed to be followed by a clear statement of what you want in a given instance (the third component). Both of these components are used in most situations when you want to be assertive.

The fourth component is the escalating one, which states the consequences (either positive or negative) resulting from your expectations or your future intentions if you deem them necessary. Like the first, this component is not always needed. However, there will be occasions when you find that its use is beneficial. It can be a very respectful way of letting other people know your future intentions openly and honestly, without surprising them later on.

Example 1

You recently purchased an appliance from a local department store. It is not functioning properly, and you would like a new one. You hate to return merchandise and often feel embarrassed, but you realize the necessity of such action in this situation. You are convinced that you do not want to take a financial loss and that you have a right to get what you pay for. So you pack up the appliance and your sales slip and go to the store. On arrival, you say to the salesperson in an assertive manner:

DESCRIPTION OF SITUATION	"I purchased this mixer a few weeks ago. It's not working properly.
EXPECTATIONS	I'd like a new one."

In this situation, there is no need to use the first component. It is not necessary to say "I know you really want to sell workable mixers." Instead, describing the situation and stating what you want are sufficient. Depending upon the salesperson's response, you may choose to escalate by using the fourth component. If your request is denied, you may want to speak with the manager about the matter.

Notice the use of "I" statements in the example, which is an important characteristic of an assertive approach, and the absence of aggressive "you" statements that place blame on the other person. The use of "I" statements indicates taking responsibility for your part in the situation, and it reduces the possibility of negativism or retaliation from the other person.

Example 2

You are in a middle management position. One of your employees is rarely on time for work. You have contemplated saying something to her about it but have been reluctant because you know about her problematic home situation. However, you have decided that her tardiness must stop. You realize that it is unfair to the other employees who get to work on time. Besides, you feel that you have a right to expect 8 hours of work for 8 hours of pay.

This morning, she came to the unit a ½ hour late. You ask the reason for her delay and then say assertively:

EMPATHIC COMPONENT	"I understand that things are difficult for you at home.
DESCRIPTION OF SITUATION	But I notice you have been late too many times.
EXPECTATIONS	It is necessary for you to be here on time from now on."

Because the employee in this example has been habitually late, you may want to escalate by using the fourth component to let her know what you plan to do if your expectations are not met:

NEGATIVE CONSEQUENCE	"If you're late again, I will document the incident, include it in

your personnel record, and report it to the supervisor."

or

POSITIVE CONSEQUENCE   "If you get here on time, we'll
all feel better about starting off
the shift in an organized way."

In the given situation, it is appropriate to use the empathic
component to show your concern, if you honestly feel concern, for
the other person's predicament. However, this need not change
your expectations that the employee should be at work on time. As
her superior, you may want to provide some additional guidance
or help her explore other alternatives to handle her difficulties at
home. Nevertheless, discussion of her home problems should be
kept to the essentials. Although they may influence her work performance, they are not your primary responsibility.

When implementing the components, it is imperative to give
purposeful consideration to what you want or to what the situation warrants and then to state that expectation clearly and concisely. In the professional situation described previously, the nursing manager wanted her subordinate to be at work on time. If you
find yourself being indecisive about desired results, take time to
solve the problem prior to practicing the assertive components. To
help clarify this in your own mind, you may want to ask yourself
"What do I really want in this situation?"

You Can Be Assertive

Successful assertions require planning and practice, especially if
assertiveness is a new behavior for you. It is unrealistic to think
that you can suddenly become assertive after years of behaving
otherwise. However, nurses in our sessions, after a very brief period
of time, have assertively made significant changes in their lives.
These events have included changing jobs, entering collegiate nursing programs, initiating divorce proceedings, and returning to professional employment. We believe that many of these people who

made pronounced alterations in their life-styles very quickly had contemplated making the changes for awhile and just needed the impetus and the "permission" that sessions on assertiveness can provide.

You can be assertive, too, in the course of daily events and to the degree you desire if:

1. You are convinced of the value of assertiveness in a given situation.
2. You feel confident enough to try.
3. You overcome whatever inhibiting factors may be present.
4. You plan and practice your approach.
5. You are persistent and do not permit yourself to be discouraged or thwarted easily.

Assertiveness is a skill that can be learned and perfected through experience. Nurses practice technical skills until they become confident of their competence. Similarly, through practice, the interpersonal skill of assertiveness can be perfected. While not all nurses may want to be assertive, we believe that those who do, can change their behavior, especially if they have the necessary guidance and support to help them.

References

Ashley, JoAnn. *Hospitals, Paternalism and the Role of the Nurse.* New York: Teachers College Press, 1976.

Berne, Eric. *Games People Play.* New York: Random House, 1964.

Bloom, Lynn, Karen Coburn, and Joan Pearlman. *The New Assertive Woman.* New York: Dell, 1975.

Dean, Patricia Geary. Toward Androgeny. *Image* 10 (1978):10–14.

Ehrenreich, Barbara, and Deirdre English. *Complaints and Disorders.* New York: Feminist Press, 1973. (a)

Ehrenreich, Barbara, and Deirdre English. *Witches, Midwives and Nurses.* New York: Feminist Press, 1973. (b)

Greenleaf, Nancy P. *The Politics of Self-Esteem.* Wakefield, Mass.: Nursing Digest/Contemporary Publication, 1978.

Grissum, Marlene, and Carol Spengler. *Womanpower and Health Care.* Boston: Little, Brown, 1976.

Heide, Wilma Scott. Nursing and Women's Liberation: A Parallel. *American Journal of Nursing* 73 (1973):824–827.

Kramer, Marlene. *Reality Shock.* St. Louis: C. V. Mosby, 1974.

Lazarus, Arnold M. Women in Behavior Therapy. In *New Psychotherapies for a Changing Society,* edited by Violet Franks and Vasanti Burtle. New York: Brunner/Mazel, 1974.

Mauksch, Ingeborg. Future of Nursing Practice. Speech delivered at Nursing East, Pennsylvania Nurses Association Summer Symposium, Lancaster, Pennsylvania, 1980.

Morgan, Marabel. *The Total Woman.* Old Tappan, N.J.: Fleming H. Revell, 1973.

2

Deciding Whether to Be Assertive

You and another registered nurse are both working with one aide on the 3:00-to-11:00 P.M. shift. One of your patients must be started on compresses immediately, and you are hurrying to begin an intravenous on him. You pass the aide in the hall and tell her to start the compresses. She says, "I'm already passing water pitchers to the other nurse's patients. You'll have to get someone else."

How would you feel? What would you say?

As the assistant director of nursing, you are responsible for staff development. You have scheduled a 6-week educational program for the critical care nurses in your setting and have planned the dates with your colleague, the assistant director for the specialty units. You have rented films and arranged for guest speakers. On the day before the program, your colleague approaches you and says, "I can't let the staff who were scheduled for your classes attend. There are too many vacations now, and we need coverage."

How would you feel? What would you say?

For the past 6 months, you have been responsible for compiling a report of decisions reached at weekly nurse audit meetings. You were told by your supervisor, who assigned you the task, that this responsibility would be passed from person to person as new individuals joined the committee. Two months ago a new member joined the group, but you are still compiling the reports.

How would you feel? What would you say?

What would you do in response to each of these situations? Even more importantly, what kinds of attitudes, beliefs, and feelings would influence your behavior? The intent of this chapter is to help you understand the various factors that influence your decision to be assertive, passive, or aggressive.

What Are the Advantages and Disadvantages of Being Assertive?

When contemplating a change in behavior, it is necessary to recognize that making the actual decision to change and the commitment to work at that change may be the most difficult part of all. It is important to consider what you will be giving up as well as what you will be gaining. Exploring some of the advantages and disadvantages of nonassertive (passive) behavior and assertive behavior can be helpful to you in deciding whether you want to change (Bloom, Coburn, and Pearlman, 1975). Our experience has shown that more nurses want to progress from passiveness to assertiveness than from aggressiveness to assertiveness; therefore, the following comparisons are made from that perspective.

For the most part, remaining passive allows an individual to avoid external conflict or overt manifestations of anger that could lead to rejection. Because the passive nurse fears rejection, she often operates by trying to "keep the peace" at all costs. Her tendency is to do whatever others want rather than initiating or taking a stand of her own, thereby avoiding responsibility. Examples of passive responses illustrating this tendency are as follows: "However you arrange the staffing is fine" and "It's not my fault that the new schedule didn't work out. It wasn't my idea." The irony of such an approach, however, is that the very outcome the passive nurse seeks to avoid—rejection—may indeed result, especially when others become intolerant of the indecisive, noncommital behavior and, consequently, avoid her.

One common advantage of passivity is that such a person is taken care of and protected by others. People may feel sorry for the passive nurse because she is "too shy" to speak up, with the result that they "take charge." "Let me do this for you" and "I'll take care of it so you won't have to bother" are welcome offers to the passive person. In addition, the praise a passive individual receives for conforming to others' expectations serves as a motivating force to perpetuate the passive behavior. "You're so easy to get along with" and "If there were more people like you, this place would be a lot better" are typical remarks made to a passive nurse who places everyone else's needs ahead of her own.

Finally, it is comfortable for a passive person to remain passive because such behavior fits a familiar pattern. Whenever one attempts to alter a well-established routine, a sense of discomfort and uneasiness ensues. It is less agonizing to the self to maintain the status quo than to accept the turbulence of change.

In summary, the advantages of nonassertive (passive) behavior are the following:

1. The avoidance of external conflict, anger, and rejection
2. The avoidance of responsibility
3. Protection by others
4. Praise for conforming to others' expectations
5. Comfort in maintaining a familiar behavior pattern

Clearly, nonassertive behavior causes certain negative consequences for an individual. Exploring and recognizing these disadvantages can help you to determine whether you want to be assertive in a given situation. Whenever you find yourself saying yes to a request that you really want to deny, you may feel internal anger or turmoil. For instance, agreeing to socialize with a friend when you would prefer to pursue your own interests for the day, or reluctantly accommodating a colleague by working on your day off, may evoke uncomfortable feelings within you. In addition, your self-respect may be reduced, and you may feel internal dishonesty because you did not have the courage to say no. The experience of lacking control over your own behavior can contribute further to lowering your self-esteem.

Behaving passively creates a climate for others to take care of you, automatically placing you in a dependent position. Of course, how others choose to take care of you will vary; some may be abusive and take advantage of your dependent position, while others may behave more charitably toward you. The point is that the passive nurse who does not take control of her own personal and work life remains powerless and vulnerable to the whims of others. Allowing others to make decisions for you is an overt manifestation of diminished self-control.

To summarize, the disadvantages of being nonassertive (passive) are as follows:

1. Inner turmoil or anger
2. Reduction of self-respect
3. Feelings of dishonesty
4. Lack of self-control
5. Dependency
6. Loss of decision-making ability

Very simply, the reverse of these disadvantages reflects the *advantages* of assertive behavior. When you speak up and communicate in an open, honest, and direct way without infringing on the rights of others, your chances increase for developing the following characteristics:

1. Inner peace, satisfaction, and comfort
2. Self-respect
3. Honesty
4. Self-control
5. Independence
6. Decision-making power and ability

Of course, it is not always possible or even necessarily in your best interest to have all these attributes exist as a result of every situation, since there are varying degrees and styles of assertiveness. In fact, there will be times when you choose to be dependent, to relinquish some control, or to delegate some of your decision-making ability to others and still be assertive.

For example, suppose that the last 6 months have been especially draining for you, and you have expended a great deal of energy managing your family and professional life. As vacation time approaches, you feel the need to be taken care of. Your husband is eager to select a vacation site and make reservations, and you do not want to examine the details. Instead, you convey your wishes in generalities: your desire for a quiet, restful vacation spot near a body of water with complete accommodations, the omission of sight-seeing tours, and a maximum of 5 hours of driving time from your home. You feel very comfortable trusting your husband to select a location and make the arrangements. In fact, you encourage him to do so.

In another instance, suppose that as the assistant director of medical nursing in a large urban hospital, you and the supervisory staff are working hard to develop a competent, reliable, and accountable group of head nurses. Although the hiring of new staff members for the medical units comes under your jurisdiction, you and the group of head nurses have agreed on the benefits of their being responsible for interviewing, hiring, and firing their own nursing personnel. You have offered your guidance and assistance as needed, and you intend to make yourself available to them.

While on the surface, it may seem in each of these situations that you are passively allowing other people to "take over" for you, in reality you are selecting a course of action for yourself with a goal in mind. In each example, you purposefully have chosen to depend on another person's selection, to relinquish control of an area in which you could have more influence, and to delegate some of your decision-making power to another. Although all the advantages of being assertive listed previously are not fulfilled in these two examples, a degree of assertiveness is maintained.

In the personal example, the wife's goal was to free herself of the details of selecting and arranging a vacation site. However, she established certain guidelines and communicated them assertively to her husband. An added benefit of choosing to remove herself from the selection and arrangement process was the message of trust she conveyed to her husband regarding his judgment.

In the professional example, the assistant director had as her goal the establishment of a responsible group of head nurses who could develop a cohesive, competent, and satisfied staff. Assertively, she communicated her willingness to trust them by fostering their own growth and independent judgment with her support.

In both situations, the initiator of the action most likely experienced internal satisfaction, self-respect, integrity, and self-control, all important hallmarks against which to measure the effectiveness and appropriateness of one's own behavior. In most instances, the attainment of these characteristics is an outgrowth of behaving assertively.

The Relationship between Assertiveness and Decision Making

While assertive behavior is important and necessary for the advancement of nursing, it should be used with discretion and good judgment. It is not always appropriate to be assertive, just as it is not always appropriate to be passive or aggressive. There are instances in which variations of these three types of behavior are appropriate and necessary.

The choice about whether to be assertive—and if so, when, to what degree, and in what manner—is related to one's decision-making ability. So often, when nurses are concerned about their inability to be assertive in a given situation, the difficulty lies in the fact that they have not made a clear decision about the situation. The fact that it is difficult to be assertive when you are ambivalent illustrates the importance of being able to make sound decisions. Decision making is deliberate and action oriented. Competence in decision making is part of being assertive, for it can provide added freedom and control over your life.

It is not surprising that many nurses have difficulty making decisions, since typical early educational and practice settings did not provide the opportunity to develop effective decision-making skills. Students traditionally experienced two extremes: Either most decisions were made for them in the form of rules, regulations, dress codes, and courses of study; or they were left prematurely in charge of clinical units to make decisions regarding patient care without the necessary instruction and support, leaving them with little confidence about their decision-making ability.

Today's nursing world demands that nurses know how to make decisions effectively. In order to do this, it is important to understand and master the steps of the decision-making process. The following steps of the decision-making process, upon which the remainder of this chapter is based, are a modification and expansion of the framework developed by Gelatt, Varenhorst, Carey, and Miller (1973):

- DEFINE THE DECISION to be made.
- Know what you want; identify your GOALS.
- Know what is important to you; identify your VALUES.
- Recognize your FEELINGS.
- Identify REALITY; examine the facts and seek new information.
- Assess the RISKS and costs of each alternative.
- Develop a plan or STRATEGY for getting what you want.
- MAKE THE DECISION.

These steps, which significantly affect one's decision to be assertive, are interrelated and do not necessarily have to be followed in the exact order given. Typically, some of the steps may be unconscious. However, by becoming increasingly aware of them, you can strive to make the entire process a more conscious one. The various steps in the decision-making process are discussed in detail in order to illustrate their interdependence and their influence on the final steps of planning strategies for action and making your decision.

Define the Decision to Be Made

One of the reasons that nurses have difficulty being assertive is that they often do not accurately define the central problem in a given situation. Clearly defining the problem is important, for solutions work only when they are applied to the right problems (Stevens, 1980). Drucker (1973) has suggested that Americans may benefit from the decision-making process used by the Japanese wherein the Japanese do not focus primarily on finding a solution to a problem but rather place more emphasis on defining the real issue or question. Sometimes related issues must be clarified and dealt with separately.

For example, refer to the three situations on the opening pages of this chapter. Besides deciding whether to be assertive, the nurse in each situation has another decision to make. In the situation with the aide, the nurse has to decide, after receiving the aide's refusal of her request, if she wants to insist that the aide put compresses on the patient. In the second situation, the decision to be made after learning about the scheduling difficulty is whether the staff development nurse still wants to offer the classes for the critical care nurses or whether she wants to cancel them temporarily or permanently. And in the third situation, the issue to be decided is whether the nurse will continue to do the reports or whether she will refuse. In each of these situations, a related issue involves the nurse's approach and whether she wants to implement her primary decision in an assertive way.

Know What You Want; Identify Your Goals

When making a conscious decision about whether to be assertive, an essential consideration should be your goal: What is it that you specifically want to accomplish? Although the need to determine your goal may seem too basic to warrant discussion, experience has shown that many individuals overlook this primary step in making a decision about whether to behave assertively. Yet it is imperative to consider your desired end result in order to progress through the steps of the decision-making process.

If the nurse's goal in the situation with the aide is specifically to communicate to the aide the importance of following directions, the nurse may choose to be firm in her rebuttal to the aide's initial refusal. If, however, her goal is simply to get the compresses done, she may ask the other nurse to help her out, or she may start them herself. In the second example, if the nurse in staff development really wants to provide critical care classes, she may explore alternatives for conducting them at another time. Finally, if the nurse responsible for compiling the report of the nurse audit meetings has a definitive goal of relinquishing that task, she might plan her strategies accordingly.

Know What Is Important to You; Identify Your Values

If it is possible to single out the most important consideration in the decision-making process as it relates to assertiveness, it is the influence of personal values. Once the issue about which a decision is to be made is defined, values impact significantly on all the other steps in the decision-making process. Values affect your goals, your feelings about yourself and others, and your ability to assess yourself and the circumstances of a situation realistically, to take risks, and ultimately to develop strategies for action and to make the decision.

For instance, if you value kindness, generosity, and concern for others, you may have positive feelings about a person who possesses these qualities; whereas if you devalue competitiveness, power, and status, you may have negative feelings about a person with these characteristics. Additionally, if you value yourself, you will be in a better position to establish limits and to be realistic regarding your involvement in situations than if you do not consider yourself valuable. Further, if your goal or desired outcome in a given situation is important and is valued highly enough, you will be more inclined to take a risk in order to obtain it; often that risk includes assertive behavior. Finally, if you value assertiveness as a way of life, you will be more likely to implement your decision in an assertive manner and to invest the time and energy necessary to develop the skills to become an assertive person.

Values and How They Relate to Assertiveness

According to Simon and Kirschenbaum (1972), every decision and action an individual takes is based either consciously or unconsciously on personal beliefs, attitudes, and values. Values constitute a set of personal beliefs and attitudes about the truth, beauty, or worth of any thought, object, or behavior (Raths, Harmin, and Simon, 1966). Values are important to human existence because they are action oriented and productive. Values are ongoing and "in progress"—in other words, they change as new and relevant data are examined. They are personal guidelines from which judgments are made and action is taken. Values provide a frame of reference and a basic comprehension of reality through which people integrate, explain, and appraise new ideas, events, and personal relationships (Uustal, 1978).

Beliefs and attitudes become values when they satisfy seven steps within the following three processes (Raths, Harmin, and Simon, 1966):

CHOOSING	1. Values must be chosen freely and not be indoctrinated.
	2. Values must be chosen from among alternatives. There must be a choice.
	3. Values must be chosen after considering the consequences of the choice.
PRIZING	4. You are proud of your choice and values.
	5. You publicly affirm your values. You actively support your stand.
ACTING	6. You make it part of your behavior. Talking about an issue but doing nothing is not acting on the value.
	7. You do it repeatedly. When you value something, you apply it to your life in many situations. (pp. 28–30)

Values, then, are those beliefs which meet all seven of these criteria. Not coincidentally, these same criteria are applicable to assertiveness. In the following list, the concept of assertiveness is substituted for the concept of values.

CHOOSING	1. Assertiveness must be chosen freely and not be indoctrinated. 2. Assertiveness must be chosen from among alternatives. There must be a choice. 3. Assertiveness must be chosen after considering the consequences of the choice.
PRIZING	4. You are proud of your choice of assertive behavior. 5. You publicly affirm your assertions. You actively support your stand.
ACTING	6. You make it part of your behavior. Talking about an issue but doing nothing is not acting assertively. 7. You do it repeatedly. When you truly integrate the principles of assertiveness, you apply them to your life in many situations.

Recently, numerous publications and workshops related to values clarification have been aimed at helping nurses understand the importance of values and their relationship to nursing practice. Values clarification is a way of discovering what is meaningful to you. Its purpose is not to indoctrinate a specific set of beliefs, since one set is not appropriate for all people, but rather to allow each nurse to discover her own values. Values clarification is the process of examining alternatives and selecting what is important and right for you (Uustal, 1978).

One way of clarifying values is through the process of "centering" (O'Neill and O'Neill, 1975). "Centering" refers to getting in touch with various aspects of yourself such as your values, feelings, needs, and goals. Through this process, you can come to know who you really are and the things that are most important to you. If previously you were unaware of these aspects of yourself, you may experience a transitional period of self-centeredness. This concentrated self-assessment phase is a necessary step in becoming assertive (Pardue, 1980).

Centering is the first step in initiating change in your own behavior. It can help you not only to find a new direction in life but also to feel confidence in yourself regardless of how your life changes or what direction you take. If you value yourself (and assertive people do value themselves), you will provide yourself with the opportunity to center. While different people use various ways to get in touch with their inner selves, the following techniques are offered as suggestions (O'Neill and O'Neill, 1975).

1. *Don't be afraid to waste time.*

If you feel that you always have to be doing something "constructive," you may have a difficult time getting in touch with yourself. We all need time to be alone with ourselves to do nothing. Within reason, "wasted time" is healthy and useful. In reality, it is not actually wasted; it is simply unstructured. Often it is in these moments that we are most open to our unconscious reservoir of creativity.

2. *Allow yourself to daydream.*

Daydreaming can be productive in helping you to center. By permitting yourself to fantasize and imagine, you can get in touch with what you want in reality. Daydreams can help to provide you with more creative, flexible ways of problem solving and can increase your motivation to reach solutions. By channeling your daydreams, you can take an assertive step in planning change in your life.

3. *Dialogue with yourself.*

Allow yourself to receive your own thoughts and feelings in

an open and honest way. Have a free-flowing dialogue with yourself in which you can examine your hurts and pains authentically,
along with your happiness and joys.

4. *Validate things with yourself.*

Ask yourself questions. Search out your own values. Identify
the priorities that are most important to you in a given situation or
specific time in your life, recognizing that these priorities may
change as you progress through life's stages. Begin to own yourself. Let your own thoughts and feelings be your guide instead of
looking to others for approval or permission. Supply your own
answers in situations by assertively saying yes when you want to
say yes and no when you want to say no (Chapter 5).

5. *Talk with others.*

The meaning of many of your feelings and experiences is
vague until you begin to talk about them. Sharing happenings
with a trustworthy person can help you to clarify beliefs and feelings, promote growth, and discover ways to change.

The process of centering helps to provide the basis from which
we can then select a course of action or direction. However, centering in and of itself is not sufficient. If a person centers exclusively
on his inner self, he can become introverted. Centering must be carried further.

The next phase is called "focusing" (O'Neill and O'Neill,
1975). "Focusing" means to concentrate your attention on one
particular thing, to make it distinct in order to clarify your relationship to it, and to become involved with it. Focusing is the process of making connections between your inner self and the external
world. Figure 1, which is used in Gestalt psychology, demon-
strates the principle of focusing. If you concentrate on the white
center section of the picture, you see a vase. The black area becomes
the background. However, if you focus on the shaded areas on either
side, you see two human profiles facing each other. The white center section then becomes the background. Obviously, you can

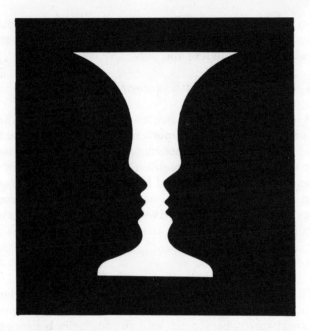

FIGURE 1. A Gestalt demonstration of focusing (from Nena O'Neill and George O'Neill, *Shifting Gears,* New York, Avon Books, 1975).

make a decision about where to place your focus. This perceptual exercise illustrates how we have a similar choice regarding our focus in daily events and life in general.

We are also free to change our focus when we choose. The nurse who decides to take a temporary leave of absence from her job to pursue an advanced degree is focusing on the value of education for her future career. Being perceptive enough to recognize that the specialty in which you are functioning is no longer satisfying to you and assertively changing to another area of nursing is focusing your efforts in a constructive way.

Often people try to focus on too many things at once and have difficulty making decisions about one focus and other. This problem is evident in newly promoted nurse managers who have trouble choosing between being "one of the gang" with their co-workers and functioning as an authority figure. Frequently, the value conflict between being well liked and getting the job done interferes with choosing a focus. Typically, when people fluctuate between options and are unable to make a choice between one focus and another, indecision and frustration result.

The processes of centering and focusing are ongoing. Like two sides of a coin, they are integral to each other. Without both, there can be no whole. Likewise, we cannot grow or change without involvement in the outside world. By opening up to things and individuals outside ourselves, we see that other people's ideas, values, and ways of doing things are different from ours. We can be challenged by such observations and subsequently reexamine and reevaluate ourselves. Our vitality and ability to grow and change exist only in our confrontation and engagement with life. Thus, the interrelated processes of centering and focusing can help us to reach the point of making a decision about how to move forward assertively and change.

What is your focus? What are your beliefs and convictions? As a nurse, where do you stand on health care issues such as euthanasia, abortion, or artificial organ transplants? How do these beliefs affect the care that you give to patients? Are you an advocate of patients' rights, national health insurance, or third-party reimbursement for nurses? What do you believe about professional autonomy, joint practice, or peer review? Your values concerning all these issues have implications not only for your clinical practice but also for your professional relationships with nursing colleagues and other health care personnel.

Identifying your values can help you to set priorities and influence your decision about when to be assertive and when not to be assertive. For example, assume that you are working on a surgical unit and on a given morning have arrived at work late because of unpredictable circumstances at home. Somehow your tardiness sets up a chain of unpleasant events on the unit, and by 10 A.M. you feel exasperated. You can tell that it is going to be one of those days!

In response to an error on your part, a particular physician, who is known for his caustic remarks, asks you sarcastically how long you have been out of school, implying that you are functioning as a fledgling nurse. With everything else that has happened on this particular morning, your tolerance is about exhausted. Although you would like to lash back, you decide that it is in your best interest to keep quiet and be nonassertive. Besides, you are extremely busy with patient care, which is your current priority. In addition, you feel that using your energy to deal with the physician's remark immediately is not a priority. However, you intend to regain your composure and, when the situation is less hectic, approach the physician assertively about his manner toward you. You have wanted to confront him for a long time, and this episode provides just the impetus you need.

The fact that values are reflected in actions can be demonstrated further by reexamining the three examples presented in the opening pages of this chapter. In response to the first situation, in which an aide refused to apply compresses as directed (stating that she was already passing water pitchers to another nurse's patients), nurses react in various ways, depending on their value systems. Those nurses who value being liked by others and who do not want to "ruffle any feathers" choose to perform both tasks themselves rather than create an uncomfortable situation with a subordinate. Obviously, this type of behavior is passive.

Others, who value authority and have no qualms about letting the aide know who is "boss," insist that the compresses be done immediately. They may make their point in an attacking, sarcastic, or demeaning way—for example, "When I tell you to do something, I want you to do it. The compresses for Mr. Jones are more important than those water pitchers. Now get them done!" While these statements may be true, the manner in which they are said and the message conveyed are aggressive.

A third group, who value both efficiency and respect, might say, "I know that you're busy with the water pitchers, but the compresses are more important right now. I'd like you to put them on Mr. Jones. I'll tell the other nurse that I've asked you to help me for the moment and that you'll get back to the water pitchers as soon as you're finished." This response is assertive and, although not essential, utilizes the empathic component of the assertive response/approach. In addition, the nurse takes responsibility for communicating the aide's change in assignment to her colleague since it was she who initiated it. Following this type of response, not only would the job get done but the aide's respect for the nurse would be enhanced.

In the second example at the beginning of the chapter, a colleague, the assistant director for the specialty units, cancelled the attendance for your staff development critical care program the day before it was to be held, citing vacations and lack of coverage as the reasons. If your commitment to present the program as scheduled was top priority and you highly valued following through with your plans exactly as they were made, you might proceed by telling your colleague firmly that since she gave you late notice when you had already rented films and arranged for speakers, the program would be held as scheduled. Further, you could state that you expect her to be sure the participants are in attendance, regardless of what measures she has to take to have them there; additionally, if they are not in attendance, you could tell her that you would speak with the director of nursing about the matter.

If, however, you have a high regard for time, money, and personal effort, your anger over the timing of her remark may prompt you to handle the situation differently. Recognizing that it would be unrealistic to attempt to hold the program the next day as scheduled, you might propose to your colleague that the two of you jointly select an alternative date, that she share the responsibility for phoning the speakers and explaining the situation, and that part of the cost for film rental come out of her budget.

On the other hand, if you have a laissez-faire attitude and you view cancellation of the program as less work for you, you may welcome unexpected "free time." Or, if getting along with this co-worker at all costs is of value to you, you may accept the last-minute change of plans passively.

As a final comparison, the third situation described at the beginning of the chapter involved an assignment given to you by your supervisor to compile a weekly report of nursing audit meetings. You had been assured that when a new member joined the group, the responsibility for the reports would be delegated to that individual, but that had not been the case. If you value authority and unquestioningly following assignments, you probably will continue to complete the reports indefinitely until either your superior or someone else initiates a change. You may be disgruntled and gripe about the task, but taking responsibility for altering it may not fit into your passive style. Or perhaps, because you value your ability to compile data and write reports, you believe that the reason the task is not being delegated to someone else is because you are doing such a good job!

In contrast to either of these beliefs, your attitude might be that your time and energy can be used more productively in another capacity. You value fairness and "taking your turn," but within reasonable limits. You believe that since another member joined the committee two months ago, it is now her turn to begin compiling the reports. You plan to communicate this fact to your supervisor in an assertive manner at the next opportunity.

As evidenced in these hypothetical examples, different values evoke different analyses and different responses to the same circumstances and situations. The more clear you are about what you believe, the better able you will be to make decisions and to choose a self-satisfying behavioral course of action congruent with those beliefs.

The Value of Respecting Others

Assertiveness, as defined in Chapter 1, includes the recognition and acceptance of other people. Specifically, the integrity of others is maintained through the use of the empathic component of the assertive response/approach. However, treating people with respect by recognizing their values and communicating to them that they are valuable does not always occur.

Many times different values can be a source of conflict. Such an example was shared by a staff nurse working in a rural community hospital. She was caring for a patient with an inoperable brain tumor who had recently returned from a nearby medical center where a complete diagnostic work-up had been done. The patient's skin was beginning to break down, and the nurse wanted an ointment ordered. But the physician refused, saying the concern was "trivial" and that the patient had "more important things" wrong with her.

Certainly, the nurse's values in this situation were different from the physician's. In discussing the incident, the nurse believed

that her assessment of the patient's skin condition was accurate
and that treatment was indicated. However, when she was confronted with the physician's roadblock, she did not know what to
do. A suggested strategy for the nurse to implement after deciding
what she wanted would be to say assertively:

EMPATHIC COMPONENT	"I realize that you are concerned with other aspects of Mrs. K's care and that excoriated skin may sound insignificant in relation to the scope of her condition.
DESCRIPTION OF SITUATION	But her discomfort is also an important consideration.
EXPECTATIONS	The area in question needs to be seen and a treatment ordered or at least a verbal order given.
POSITIVE CONSEQUENCES	If her skin is taken care of now, the chances will be better of preventing further skin deterioration later on."

By using the empathic component of the assertive response/
approach, the nurse can communicate respect for the physician
and her understanding of his values while also stating her own
values and expectations clearly.

Acceptance of another person's values, manner of relating, or
performance of a task when these are different from our own is
sometimes difficult. Yet others have a right to be different. For example, how do you treat a co-worker who chooses to spend her
available time talking with patients because she values that area
of her job more than performing routine nonclinical tasks on the
unit? Or how do you treat the subordinate who will not relinquish
attending a particular sport event with her family to work a double
shift or make a presentation at a special meeting? Or what about
the nurse who works "only" part time or the one who chooses not
to obtain academic credentials?

Are these nurses ostracized because their values and choices are different from the norm? Is it not possible that a nurse who chooses to work intermittently during her childbearing years, or who chooses to place nursing second in priority to family responsibilities or other pleasures in life, or who chooses either not to obtain an academic degree or to obtain one in a nonnursing discipline can also make a meaningful and valuable contribution, especially if she is valued?

Evidence of devaluing each other can be seen between shifts on a given unit or between the general hospital units and the specialty units, where one group may act superior to another. We must not undermine those colleagues who select a slightly different route from the one we arbitrarily decide to be the best or whose values and choices are different from our own. Even though we may disagree with each other, we can learn to treat one another with respect and dignity. We teach respect and dignity for patients and patients' values—why not respect for nurses and nurses' values?

The assertive nurse recognizes that she cannot control other people's choices. She assumes responsibility for making her own decisions and for controlling her own behavior. She knows that just as she has the right to make her own choices assertively, so do her nursing colleagues.

Expecting to Be Valued

In addition to communicating respect and value to others, it is important to expect others to value you. This expectation can be accomplished by valuing yourself. In fact, there is considerable evidence to support the relationship between self-acceptance, acceptance of others, and acceptance by others (Hamachek, 1971; Johnson, 1972). People who are self-accepting are usually more accepting of others and, consequently, are accepted in return. In other words, if you value yourself, you are likely to value others, and others will reciprocate by valuing you. Conversely, if you devalue yourself, you are likely to devalue others, and they are likely to reciprocate by devaluing you.

These self-fulfilling prophecies are actually confirmed as a result of your behavior (Johnson, 1972). For example, Kathy, a class participant, explained how she was ultimately valued by her head nurse. She related an incident in which she had been working on the weekend caring for a terminally ill patient with chronic lung disease. Because he had been on her unit a number of times, she was well acquainted with his circumstances and knew that neither the patient nor his family wanted resuscitation. Thus, when an episode occurred necessitating such a decision, Kathy respected their wishes. However, the head nurse, who was not working at the time, disagreed strongly with this approach and let her beliefs be known. When she returned on Monday morning and learned of the weekend happenings, she aggressively berated and belittled Kathy in front of the other staff. Kathy was convinced of the appropriateness of her actions and managed to respond assertively to the verbal attack. She expressed her anger and frustration appropriately to the head nurse while maintaining the firmness of her convictions.

The situation clearly represented a value conflict. At the time of the aggressive outburst, Kathy certainly did not feel valued by her boss, but she felt confident enough about her beliefs to uphold them and to take responsibility for her actions. Through her manner, she conveyed her expectation to be treated with respect. Later she reported that the head nurse was more personable with her and did indeed treat her with added respect. Kathy's original expectations were confirmed. As an outgrowth of such expectations, one can build good relationships and, consequently, successful assertions.

In contrast to Kathy, other nurses repeatedly relate episodes in which they have difficulty maintaining self-respect; instead, they accept devaluing comments from others. In a study of the causes of burn-out, such nurses are reported to feel the greatest amount of stress from patients, physicians, or administrators who do not respect their judgment or value (Johnson, 1980). In fact, they not only feel devalued but often feel actively downtrodden and belittled. Typically, nurses receive (and permit themselves to receive) the brunt of other health professionals' omission of care. Although a multitude of examples of this type have been shared with us by class participants, only a few are included here.

Example: Devalued by patient—physician's negligence. The clinic physician is 2 hours late. Patients are upset and angry. They take out their frustrations on the nurse but are "meek and mild" when the doctor finally arrives.

The assertive nurse helps the patients to express their annoyance to the physician who was responsible for the delay in treatment.

Example: Devalued by family—x-ray's negligence. The x-ray department refuses to work a few minutes overtime to accommodate a pediatric patient. Consequently, the urinary catheter is left in place needlessly all night. The child and parents are upset, and the nurse receives belittling comments about the inconsiderate behavior of the hospital staff.

The assertive nurse supports the parents in expressing their feelings directly to the x-ray department the following day when the x-ray is finally taken. Or, when the nurse receives the phone message that the x-ray department is not willing to be detained, she can tell that department to "hold," bring one of the child's parents to the phone, and have x-ray explain the circumstances directly to the parent.

Example: Devalued by physician—faulty equipment. While in the patient's room, the physician plugs in the cauterizing equipment. It does not work. He becomes verbally abusive to the nurse, slings the equipment across the room, and stomps out.

The assertive nurse does not make an apologetic remark to the patient on the doctor's behalf but rather verbalizes what has occurred. "Obviously Dr. Jones is upset with the defective equipment. I'll look into the possibility of getting it replaced and will let you know shortly if you will still be cauterized." Meanwhile, to the physician, the nurse expresses her angry feelings in an assertive way and keeps to the issue at hand—that is, the cauterization of the patient: "I do not appreciate the insults that were made to me about the faulty cauterizing equipment. It is impossible for me to prevent equipment breakdown at any given moment, and I will not accept being berated about something over which I have no control. If you are still interested in cauterizing the patient, I will have the unit clerk phone another floor for a replacement."

Example: Devalued by physician—laboratory's negligence.
A stool specimen was ordered a number of days ago. It was sent to
the laboratory immediately, but the results are not on the chart.
The physician screams at the nurse on duty for her neglect.

In a strong, convincing manner, the assertive nurse indicates
that the specimen was sent, verifies it by showing the physician
the documentation, and suggests that he phone the laboratory to
verbalize his complaints.

Example: Devalued by nursing superior—lack of administrative support. A nursing staff development director has become
progressively discouraged about the minimal respect the nursing
staff receives in her setting and about its lack of support and advancement within her system. Furthermore, the rewards she receives from her immediate superior, the nursing director, are rare.
When she does an outstanding job, it is hardly noticed. To make
matters worse, she has overheard her boss say, "Well, if Elaine is
dissatisfied and unhappy here, perhaps she'd better leave. I have a
whole list of people on file who would welcome that position."

The assertive nurse would weigh carefully the pros and cons
of her current position while considering the circumstances of her
personal life situation and sizing up the realistic opportunities for
another job. She could try actively to improve her work situation
by making an informed decision about ways to advance her professional career instead of passively remaining a victim of the circumstances.

Discussion of examples. Although other examples could be
cited in which nurses are valued, in reality there are probably a
greater number of instances in which nurses are devalued by others. Why do you suppose nurses permit such happenings to occur
continuously without asserting themselves by setting limits,
speaking up, or initiating positive preventive action? Is it not time
to internalize the belief that no one can make us feel inferior without our consent—and to make some decisions to change our professional image both as individuals and as collective members of the
nursing profession? We can begin to do this by developing self-respect.

The Value of Self-Respect

Self-respect means to hold oneself in esteem and to consider oneself with dignity. The desire for self-esteem is thought to be an individual's most basic drive. What we really want more than anything else in the world is the realization that we are worthy persons (Schuller, 1980). Those people who have a high regard for themselves are said to be self-accepting (Johnson, 1972).

According to Hamachek (1971), a person who has a strong self-accepting attitude possesses the following characteristics (adapted from Johnson, 1972, pp. 144–145), all of which are in harmony with the nurse who behaves assertively:

1. She has a firm belief in certain values and principles which are upheld even in the face of strong group opinion. She is secure enough to modify these values, however, if new evidence or experience warrants it.

2. She acts on her own best judgment without feeling excessively guilty or regretting her actions even if others disapprove.

3. She does not spend undue time worrying about the past, the future, or the present.

4. She is confident of her ability to deal with problems, including failure and setbacks.

5. She feels equal to others as a person, regardless of their differences in abilities, family backgrounds, or attitudes.

6. She views herself as a person of interest and value to others, especially to those with whom she chooses to associate.

7. She can accept praise without pretending to be modest and compliments without feeling guilty.

8. She resists the efforts of others to dominate her.

9. She admits to herself and others that she possesses a wide range of feelings—including love, anger, sadness, joy, resentment, and acceptance.

10. She genuinely enjoys herself in a variety of activities in-

volving work, play, creative expression, companionship, and loafing.

11. She is sensitive to the needs of others, to accepted social customs, and especially to the idea that she will not advance herself at the expense of others.

Carol, a coronary care nurse, illustrates many of these characteristics in the following episode: During the course of a particular shift, she determined that the pacemaker in one of her patients was functioning improperly. When she reported this fact to the patient's cardiologist, he responded by saying that there was nothing he could do about it and that she would have to "say her prayers." After documenting the incident and informing her supervisor of the circumstances as well as her intended action, she used her own initiative to call the cardiovascular surgeon, who, after consulting with the cardiologist, proceeded to replace the pacemaker. Carol was confident of her nursing ability and firm in her conviction to act in the patient's behalf. She believed that she was acting within her rights and responsibilities as a professional nurse. Considering herself an equal member of the health team, she felt no hesitancy to proceed and certainly did not let the initial response of the attending cardiologist impede her action. She let her own beliefs and judgment be her guide.

Acting on what you think and feel, and not permitting your actions to be dominated by others does not mean, though, that you should not collaborate or ask for feedback or information from others. On the contrary, considering other people's ideas and feelings can provide valuable input for your own decision making. Listening to others and taking their opinions into consideration is not the same thing as needing their approval, however. Needing approval means giving someone else power and control over you and, in nursing, over your nursing practice. A request for feedback, on the other hand, has the purpose of gathering information which then can be balanced against your own needs and values.

In contrast to the nurse just described, many nurses have difficulty being assertive because, according to Pardue (1980), they do not see themselves as valuable and feel they are less important than physicians, nurses who are better prepared educationally, or nurses with many years of experience. Self-depreciating comparative evaluations can paralyze the nurse with self-doubt. Are you such a nurse? What do you think of yourself? Do you have self-respect? Do you consider yourself important enough to give to yourself daily—by doing something that you particularly like or can benefit from? By giving to yourself, you will be in a better position and will have more energy to give to others. Very simply, a worthwhile guideline to follow is to do what you value and value what you do (Raths, Harmin, and Simon, 1966).

One's self-concept—which is a composite of beliefs, attitudes, and feelings you have about yourself—is an influential factor in making decisions, including the decision to be assertive. One way to enhance your self-concept is to "self-disclose." To self-disclose means to share with another person your honest perceptions and feelings about events that have just taken place or something that has been said or done. It involves revealing your reactions in an open, authentic, and appropriate way while also communicating your willingness to accept the other person's self-disclosure. Self-disclosure is a necessary and important part of assertiveness. It is implicit in the second step of the components of the assertive response/approach introduced in Chapter 1.

There is evidence to indicate positive effects of self-disclosure on interpersonal relationships (Johnson, 1972). However, just as it is not appropriate to be assertive in all situations, it is not always appropriate to be self-disclosing. If you know from past experience that the other person is untrustworthy or tends to misinterpret or overreact to your openness, you may choose not to self-disclose. Nevertheless, in most cases, self-disclosure can be a positive way of letting others know you and allowing yourself to experience acceptance by them since people are more inclined to accept and value individuals they know rather than those they do not know.

As you receive positive feedback from others as a result of self-disclosing, your self-esteem will increase. By discovering that you are liked for who you are, you can begin to feel that you are truly a valuable person worthy of respect. In summary, it is much easier to be decisive and to enact your decisions in an assertive manner when you feel confident of your own self-worth and value.

Recognize Your Feelings

Like values, feelings also play a significant role in influencing the decisions we make, including decisions to behave in a certain way. Although society in general tends to view feelings as a hindrance because feelings are considered irrational, illogical, and subjective, in reality one's interpersonal effectiveness and decision-making ability can increase when all the relevant information is considered, including feelings.

Feelings are a normal, natural, and expected part of being human. Their expression is psychologically healthy. The capacity to feel is as much a part of being a person as the capacity to think and reason. The ability to experience and express feelings can be rewarding and highly constructive because it is through their expression that close relationships are built and maintained. Yet, the way we express feelings and emotions is perhaps the most frequent source of difficulty in interpersonal relationships. Problems arise not because we have feelings but because we attempt to repress, distort, or disguise them (Johnson, 1972). It is important to realize that feelings grow and evolve. They are not stagnant or unalterable but, instead, change with varying circumstances and relationships. Furthermore, different people have different feelings about the same situation.

As an illustration, refer again to the situations on the first pages of this chapter. If you were the nurse in the first example, what would your feelings be when the aide tells you that she cannot accommodate your request to begin the compresses because she is already passing water pitchers to another nurse's patients? Some nurses would be angry, others would feel "hurt," and still others would be unable to identify any specific feeling, although they know that they would take action in terms of giving a firm directive to the aide. How would you feel?

In the second situation, nurses' feelings vary from being angry in response to a colleague's renege about sending participants to the planned critical care course to fear of retaliation from the scheduled speakers and the audiovisual department. Others can understand the staffing problem and, even though the notice was received late, would accept the situation. What would your feelings be?

Most nurses express feelings of being "used" and "taken advantage of" as a result of imagining themselves in the third situation, in which the task of compiling a nursing audit report was not passed on to the newest member of the group. However, others feel pleased, believing that the continuing assignment must mean they are doing a good job. How would you feel?

As a result of analyzing the various feelings that these situations can evoke, are you able to see how some feelings can provide a stimulus for deciding to be assertive while others may precipitate either passive or aggressive behavior?

A particularly difficult situation for many people to handle is embarrassment in front of others. Fran, a staff nurse, found herself in just that kind of circumstance. She was in the nurses' station taking off orders from patients' charts. The room was filled with personnel, including students and residents. When she came across one particular order that was difficult to read, she questioned the physician who had written it and asked him to clarify the order. He became irate and shouted loudly that Fran was illiterate. She felt hurt and devastated to be embarrassed in front of so many people and could not utter a sound; it was all she could do to keep from crying. Obviously, her feelings directly influenced her passive behavior. Someone else in the same situation may have felt angry enough to retaliate with aggression. How would your feelings have influenced your behavior?

Recognizing feelings is foreign for some people, and accepting ownership of them is even more difficult. Yet feelings that are unrecognized, unaccepted, and unresolved can affect one's perception of events and cause distortions in interpersonal situations. It is not unusual for people to reject a good idea when it comes from a person they dislike or to behave aggressively for the same reason. On the other hand, recognition, acceptance, and control of one's feelings can be positive factors in stimulating assertive behavior.

Janet, a class participant, shared how she was able to identify her feelings, control them, and behave in an assertive manner with her boss. As one of four assistant directors of nursing, she was expected to take a turn working holidays. On one occasion when she walked into the nursing office, the secretary presented her with a sign-up list of various holidays for the year. Each of the assistant directors was to designate the one holiday she would be willing to work. However, when Janet received the list, all the holidays were accounted for except Christmas. She felt "set up" and could feel herself getting angry. Recognizing this fact, she decided not to ventilate her feelings on the secretary but rather to control them and determine who had initiated circulation of the list. The secretary verified that it had been the director of nursing. Janet did not sign her name but, at an appropriate time, took the list with her to discuss the situation assertively with her boss.

By becoming more aware of feelings and accepting them as natural, you will be able to use them as a potentially constructive part of the decision-making process. Examine your behavior closely and try to become consciously aware of the extent to which your feelings influence the decisions you make. As a result, you should gain insight that will contribute to your decision about whether and when to be assertive.

Identify Reality; Examine Facts and Seek New Information

Recognizing your feelings and accepting yourself as a worthwhile, valuable person can help to provide you with the impetus to be assertive. However, competency in decision making—including decisions to be assertive—depends largely on your ability to implement another step in the decision-making process: assessing yourself and the situation realistically and utilizing resources.

A nurse named Jane, who was the educational coordinator of a critical care unit in a large federally operated hospital, illustrated the ability to evaluate a situation realistically. She was on the unit when a staff surgeon who was making rounds discovered that the chest tube on one of the patients was detached. Immediately he became irritated and angry with the nurses because the chest tube was detached. In a calm, assertive manner, Jane pointed out the reality of the situation, which was that a number of people had been in and out of the room checking on the patient that afternoon, including residents and medical students who also could have detected the detached chest tube. When confronted in this way, the physician stopped short, concurred with her remark, and then added, "I guess it could also have been the way I put on the tape." Jane's response to the physician's outburst reflected not only her belief in the value and competence of herself and the other nurses on the unit but also her ability to communicate the reality of the situation.

In addition to evaluating situations realistically, it is also important to assess your own personal strengths and weaknesses in a realistic manner. Through identifying your strengths, you can increase your regard for yourself and, consequently, increase your self-acceptance and your chances of being successfully assertive. Besides, you may explore and develop your potential strengths, intensify your existing ones by practicing them, and restructure weaknesses into strengths. Interestingly enough, the ability to recognize your weaknesses and consider yourself valuable enough to improve them can be one of your greatest strengths. An essential part of your decision making is not only to recognize your ability but also to accept your limitations. Knowing when and how to seek information or guidance from another person and to utilize additional resources can supply a basis for making sound decisions.

Some nurses do not realize that it is permissible to set realistic limits on others as well as themselves. An example of such a nurse is Caroline, a school nurse who enjoyed her job except for the extensive contact she had with one of the school guidance counselors. The guidance counselor had numerous psychosocial problems for which she sought Caroline's help. He had been to a number of health professionals but claimed that none of them was beneficial to him. Although it was part of Caroline's job to provide health care to school personnel as well as students, the guidance counselor occupied so much of Caroline's time that she had difficulty completing her other work. Caroline regretted the extent to which she had become involved with this man and admitted feeling that she was "in over her head" but did not know what to do about it.

Another nurse, Denise, worked in a small rural community hospital where most of the staff knew each other as neighbors. For weeks, she had been working with an emotionally disturbed practical nurse whose professional competence progressively deteriorated. Denise found herself doing much more than her share of the work. In fact, for days she was doing two jobs instead of one. Denise was reluctant, though, to report the situation because her coworker's husband was a local cardiologist for whom Denise's sister worked. Denise felt that if she called the practical nurse's poor health and work performance to the attention of the nursing administration, her sister's job might suffer.

In each of these situations, the nurse should have assessed the situation realistically by determining the facts and then should have set limits assertively. Analyzing the facts and gathering additional information when necessary can help you to identify possible strategies for action. If Caroline had originally budgeted her time more effectively between the guidance counselor and the other aspects of her job, and if she had recognized her own limitations, the situation may not have gotten out of control. If she had realized that the guidance counselor's problems were beyond her professional capabilities, she could have suggested the resources of a mental health agency. Also, she could have discussed the situation directly with the guidance counselor, shared responsibility for their current relationship, and established limits for the future.

Drucker (1973) and Stevens (1980) both caution the decision maker to separate facts from interpretations or opinions and, instead of relying on second-hand or single-source information, to seek information from the original source, if possible, and from a variety of sources, when appropriate. Instead of assuming that her sister's job would suffer if she reported the incompetent practical nurse with whom she worked, Denise should have focused on the reality of the situation. The facts were that Denise was being paid to perform one job, not two, and that patients were entitled to receive safe, competent nursing care. Denise could have sought information from a variety of sources regarding the nursing administration's possible reaction to information about the practical nurse's poor health and work performance. Also, she could have chosen to confront the practical nurse and/or the nursing administration about the situation and set limits regarding her own job performance. Of course, confronting others with reality is sometimes risky because we cannot control how others will respond to the confrontation. The element of risk is an important factor when considering alternative action plans. This brings us to the next step in the decision-making process.

Assess the Risks and Costs of Each Alternative

When making a conscious decision about whether to be assertive, the consequences of your decision must be considered. Two basic questions you may find helpful to ask yourself in this regard are the following: (*a*) If there is a possibility of negative consequences as a result of my assertion, am I willing and able to take the risk? and (*b*) If I am assertive, what is the worst possible thing that could happen?

Because of their financial situations, personal competencies, or circumstances, some individuals are in a better position than others to accept risk. Similarly, some people can handle the "worst possible" situation better than others. In a given instance, perhaps the worst thing that could happen is that you do not get what you want. Could you live with that result? If so, the risk may be worth taking. By determining whether you can accept the worst possible consequence, while not dwelling unnecessarily on it, you are more likely to be able to act assertively because you will realize that every other possible consequence of your behavior is less risky than the worst alternative.

When initially testing out assertive skills, it is wise to begin in low-risk situations, especially if assertive behavior is somewhat foreign to you. In order for your confidence to increase, it is critical to experience successful results early. Most people feel less threatened in low-risk situations because success is likely to occur. A good low-risk place to begin is with people in whom you have no personal investment or in situations in which the stakes are not high. For example, consider the following: returning low-cost merchandise to the store, expressing dissatisfaction with the food at a restaurant and requesting an alternative selection or a price modification, or communicating your desire for an itemized bill and thorough explanation of the services rendered on a home appliance. If such assertions do not pay off by providing you with what you want, usually there is little to lose and, consequently, less risk than in situations where the stakes are higher or in personal relationships such as those between people at work, family, friends, or loved ones.

When planning to enact a high-risk assertion, especially in the work setting, in addition to perhaps not getting what you want, you also should consider the possibility of any of the following results:

1. Subsequent relationships might be strained.
2. You might pay a price in terms of retaliatory action.
3. You might lose your job.

If these possibilities exist realistically, certainly you should give careful thought to whether you want to take a particular risk. For example, if you are the type of nurse who cannot tolerate others being aloof or distant with you and there is a strong likelihood of that happening as a result of your assertion, you may opt to be nonassertive. On the other hand, another nurse whose commitment to the attainment of her goal is of the highest priority may be willing to accept or work to change the less favorable interpersonal relationships that might result.

With regard to retaliation, possible unfavorable outcomes must be evaluated. A requested day off or vacation week may not be honored; your performance appraisal or salary increment may be affected adversely; the resources you need in terms of staff, equipment, or supplies may be withheld; even worse, attempts may be made to destroy your reputation or to ostracize you from certain groups. In anticipation of such occurrences, some nurses may choose not to risk being assertive, while others may feel confident that they can handle such consequences.

When the realistic possibility of job dismissal exists, it is necessary to consider your personal circumstances before risking such an outcome. How financially dependent are you on your current job? In reality, could you acquire another position? Are you dependent on a favorable reference from your current employer? What are your marketable skills? Are you limited to a given geographical area? What would a termination do to your sense of self-worth? Although actual job dismissal occurs infrequently, the possibility must be weighed carefully.

The following experience illustrates some of the high-risk possibilities previously discussed. Carl, a cardiovascular surgeon responsible for the medical care in the coronary intensive care unit in a large hospital, was an aggressive, autocratic individual who, because of his clinical competence, had the highest number of cardiovascular surgical patients in the facility. Consequently, he enjoyed a great deal of prestige. He not only exercised his authority with patients and personnel throughout the hospital but also attempted abrasively to control the nursing staff in the coronary intensive care unit.

As a new head nurse trying to establish her role and responsibility regarding the nursing management of the unit, Linda had experienced several incidents in which Carl inappropriately attacked the staff about relatively minor items such as charts being in the wrong place. Whenever Linda offered an explanation (for example, "We've been very busy, and keeping the charts in order wasn't one of our priorities at the moment"), Carl's tyranny would continue. More often than not, he was accusatory and demeaning. On one such occasion, he mentioned that Linda ought to hire an assistant head nurse if she could not handle her job alone. While she said nothing at the time, she reported later that she had been hurt and angered by the remark.

Whenever she mustered up enough courage to speak out and set limits on Carl's abusive behavior, she noticed that he treated her in a cold and distant manner, avoiding contact with her as much as possible while relating in an extremely friendly, accommodating way with her staff members. Indeed, Linda was "paying the price" for her assertive attempts.

In discussing her relationship with this physician, it was clear that Linda was very firm in her conviction to differentiate their roles and responsibilities. She saw herself as responsible for the "nursing" management of the unit; and him, for the "medical" regime. Of course, she realized that this distinction did not preclude the integration and dovetailing of their responsibilities. Her commitment to implement this belief was a strong one; however, she needed help with the mechanics of succeeding in an appropriate, respectful way in order to promote mutual respect.

Inasmuch as Linda's isolated attempts at being assertive with Carl were not accomplishing the desired results, she initiated a meeting with him to discuss the nursing and medical management of the unit and how they might work together more efficiently. Importantly, she explored the possibility of serious adverse consequences such as losing her job if her positive attempts were not interpreted accurately or if Carl indeed wanted to manage both the nursing and medical care of the unit and would look unfavorably upon a nurse eager to function more autonomously. In reality, he had a great deal of power and prestige in the facility, and Linda recognized the possibility of him using his position to her disadvantage. Nevertheless, she decided she was willing to take the risk of losing her newly acquired position because she wanted to function with Carl rather than under him.

What were Linda's chances of being supported by her boss and nursing administration? How much influence would the nursing administration have with the medical department if the problem went to that level? Linda felt that she could expect strong support from her superiors because they had always encouraged her to make decisions to promote nursing and quality patient care. In fact, when she was offered the position of head nurse, she was reminded of her competence and told that nursing administration felt she could meet the challenge of her new job and that she would be supported in that endeavor. She informed her superiors of the meeting scheduled with Carl and its possible outcome.

When making the arrangements to schedule a mutually convenient meeting time with Carl, Linda specified her desire for it to be held in a private conference room with approximately a ½ hour duration time. She prepared well for the session, identifying in advance the specific goals that she wanted to accomplish: (a) clarity and mutual agreement regarding their roles and responsibilities and (b) respectful behavior from Carl toward her and the rest of the nursing staff.

In order to accomplish her first goal, mutual agreement regarding the clarity of roles and responsibilities, Linda developed a strategy for action. A number of times, she rehearsed her opening assertive statements, utilizing the components of the assertive response/approach:

EMPATHIC COMPONENT

"I know that you feel very strongly about your beliefs regarding the way a coronary care unit should be run.

DESCRIPTION OF FEELINGS AND SITUATION

I'm feeling that I have little authority and responsibility for the unit and that everything should be done your way.

EXPECTATIONS

Since I am the head nurse, I want to manage the nursing staff and nursing care of the unit. Sometimes the way I choose to do that job is different from the way you think it ought to be done.

POSITIVE CONSEQUENCE

If we can reach some agreement about our joint responsibilities, the unit will operate more efficiently and, hopefully, the patients will receive better care."

With regard to her second objective, respectful behavior toward the head nurse and her staff, Linda formulated this approach:

EMPATHIC COMPONENT

"I know that you are under pressure and that your position as a cardiovascular surgeon carries with it a lot of responsibility.

DESCRIPTION OF FEELINGS AND SITUATION

The staff and I feel that often we receive the brunt of that

	pressure in terms of your derogatory and abrasive remarks.
EXPECTATIONS	We have no objections to constructive criticism, but we want the demeaning comments to stop.
POSITIVE CONSEQUENCES	If you will let us know what you're thinking in a more acceptable manner, our respect for you will increase."

Linda was very pleased by the results of her discussion with Carl because she felt that her assertions had opened the door to a more collaborative working relationship between them. Certain problems still needed to be solved, but she knew that she had laid the groundwork for promoting more satisfying interactions in the future.

As illustrated by the preceding examples, some situations are riskier than others. Thus, you must decide how much risk you are willing to take and how assertive you want to be.

As with the other steps in the decision-making process, values, goals, and feelings play a particularly important role in risk taking. A decision maker is more willing to take greater risks if the outcome is highly valued (Gelatt, Varenhorst, and Carey, 1972). How much risk you take can be related to how important a particular result is to you. Ironically, some people seem drawn to goals that are difficult to obtain. For such individuals, low probability equates with high desirability—and high risk. For certain nurses, this kind of challenge may mean the acquisition of a top management position, a political office, an advanced degree, or an independent practice.

Again we see the importance of the nurse-decision maker clearly defining her values. Too often nurses passively assume the values of others or accept values that have been thrust upon them. It is difficult to take risks about something that you do not value personally. Further, the courage to risk comes from the belief that your values are worthy (Viscott, 1977). Considering your values as worthy is part of your self-esteem. If you do not think highly of yourself, likewise you will not think highly enough of your values to risk for them.

Emotions also influence your ability to risk, particularly in the area of estimating risk. Sometimes an individual wants something to be true so much that he overestimates or underestimates reality. Just as a personal bias can cause parents to overestimate their child's intellectual or athletic ability, so might it cause nurses to underestimate their individual or collective power within a setting and, consequently, the amount of risk involved.

One important emotion, fear, is very influential in choosing a risky alternative. Fearful people tend to take either very high risks (to overcompensate for the fear) or very low risks, while more confident individuals are inclined to take intermediate risks (Gelatt, Varenhorst, and Carey, 1972). Fear of the unknown and your ability to deal with it can seriously impede taking a risk, especially when you consider that the outcomes of all alternatives cannot be predicted (Stevens, 1980). Confidence in your ability to deal with the outcome, whatever it may be, will reinforce risk taking.

Risk-taking behavior is learned just as values are learned. Because of different experiences, training, and interests, people differ on how much risk they are willing to take. One person may like to "take a chance," while another wants to "play it safe." Every person develops his own risk-taking style. Thus, there is no definitive "right" or "wrong" degree of risk-taking behavior. It is important to understand yourself as a risk taker and to gather as much objective data as you can about the probability of outcomes and risks involved in each situation in order to make the wisest decisions.

Typically, nurses do not take risks easily. In addition to possible reasons related to values, goals, and feelings just discussed, nurses' hesitancy to take risks probably is related to the fact that most nurses are women. Men and women perceive risks differently (Hennig and Jardim, 1976): Men see risk as a balance, a loss or a gain, affecting the future; women see risk as entirely negative and affecting the present. These perceptions dramatically affect if and how women and nurses take risks.

Additionally, nurses have not been rewarded or reinforced for being adventurous or for taking risks. Kelly (1978) points out that men have developed networks that ensure support for taking risks. Potential nurse-risk takers have no such back-up. Too often a nurse who has taken a high risk and failed does not have a supportive colleague assuring her that it was worth the effort and that the results might be better next time.

Accepting this information helps us to understand the need to learn to be better risk takers. Developing assertive techniques can help because assertive people are self-confident and not unduly afraid of making a mistake or failing. For this reason, assertive people are more apt to take risks. Nurses can adapt the broader principles of decision making and problem solving to becoming better risk takers. Viscott's (1977) dos and don'ts of risking encompass both of these processes:

DO	Have a goal.
	Ask questions.
	Know your limits.
	Make a timetable.
DON'T	Be unrealistic.
	Count on being 100% successful.
	Rush.
	Risk just to prove yourself.
	Blame others for your failure.

Nurses have much to gain personally and professionally from taking risks because most things you really want in life involve taking a risk. Risking is required to develop power as an individual and as a profession (Viscott, 1977). Assertive nurses will risk! Additionally, they will give forethought to the development of action plans to promote positive results, thus making the risk worthwhile.

Develop a Plan or Strategy for Getting What You Want

Unfortunately, many nurses do not talk about wanting something or defining ways to go about obtaining a goal. Often they are uncomfortable talking about strategies: "It's just not nice." This may be reflective of a hesitancy to seek and accept power. Importantly, deciding on an assertive approach and developing assertive skills will help nurses to change this attitude and, ultimately, their behavior.

Recognize that you have a choice of several different ways to get what you want. Because different strategies work for different people and for different problems, it is helpful to pattern yourself to think in terms of a variety of strategies. A nurse-researcher named Peg, who believed she was currently underpaid, did just that. She was employed in a large metropolitan acute care facility, doing research under the direction of a medical department chief. She had done an outstanding job in their joint research endeavor, had published, and had presented their findings at a number of clinical conferences. Once these accomplishments were to her credit, she believed the time was right for her to receive a higher salary. In order to obtain this goal, she considered three strategies:

STRATEGY 1   She could look elsewhere for a higher-paying position and resign from her present job.

STRATEGY 2   She could continue in her present position while "moonlighting" on the side by occasionally hiring herself out to other facilities as a nursing research consultant.

STRATEGY 3   She could ask her present boss for a salary increment and additional fringe benefits.

After considering various aspects of these strategies, including the risks involved in each, Peg favored Strategy 3. However, before making a definite decision, she planned more specifically how she could approach her boss. Planning the details of a strategy in advance can help an individual to determine whether the strategy is realistic and to anticipate possible consequences. Initially, Peg checked into the funding sources and found that money was available to meet her request. Her working relationship with her boss was excellent, and she was well respected by him. She also believed in her own worth and value, and felt confident of her ability as a nurse researcher and well deserving of the requested benefits. Given all these factors, she felt comfortable with her plans to implement the following assertive approach with her boss as a method for getting what she wanted.

DESCRIPTION OF FEELINGS AND SITUATION	"I'm really feeling good about the way our research is going and the part I've played in it. Considering the accomplishments and the time and effort I've put in, I feel that I deserve a salary increase with an additional vacation week.
EXPECTATIONS	I would like $200 more per month and a second week of paid vacation time.
POSITIVE CONSEQUENCES	By receiving these benefits, I will feel well compensated for my efforts."

Unfortunately, most employers in health care settings do not freely offer rewards. Realizing this fact, Peg knew the importance of asking for what she wanted. She was hoping for acceptance of the total benefit package as she presented it. However, she was realistic enough to plan how she would respond if her request was not granted. She decided on the minimum compensation that she would accept (that is, the "bottom line"), thereby building in some room for negotiation. She planned to accept no less than a $150 increment and the extra vacation time. She was prepared to resign if an acceptable form of her request was not forthcoming. Her strategies for obtaining her goal were developed. Would she make the decision to implement them?

Make the Decision

Making the decision is that point at which all of the thought becomes action (Stevens, 1980). Competency in decision making involves using all the previous described steps in the decision-making
process to choose the best alternative for you, considering the
"probable" outcomes. Notice the mention of "probable" outcomes, for an assertive nurse can control her decision but not all
the possible outcomes. It is possible to make a satisfactory decision but to have an undesirable outcome because sometimes there
are circumstances beyond an individual's control. For example,
the nurse-researcher interested in obtaining a higher salary may
have chosen to approach her boss assertively about the subject
and received his approval for her request. Six months later she
may have learned that funding sources were cut, requiring a reduction in salaries. Given the information she had at the time, she
made a good decision. However, eventually an undesirable outcome could occur.

The assertive nurse-decision maker does not chastise herself
for an unfavorable outcome; instead, she feels good that at the
time she made the best decision she could. Assertive decision making is similar to other types of assertive behavior. No one can
promise you a guaranteed success, but chances are you will feel
good about your role in the process.

Often the decision to change behavior is the most difficult
choice of all. In making this decision, it may be helpful for you to
review the advantages and disadvantages of being assertive discussed at the beginning of this chapter. What do you have to gain
or lose by relinquishing your usual nonassertive behavior? Do the
gains outweigh the losses? What are the risks involved? What are
your feelings about yourself, and what is the reality of your circumstances? You might also want to ask yourself: What are my short-
and long-term goals? Can assertiveness be an effective strategy to
help me attain them? Do I value change, assertiveness, and myself
enough to exert the effort necessary to alter my behavior?

Unquestionably, the manner of implementing a decision is
just as important as making it since implementation style can influence the outcome of a decision. In other words, once the decision

to be assertive is made, the manner in which the nurse enacts her assertion is crucial to its success. These implementation techniques are discussed in subsequent chapters.

If you are dissatisfied in certain respects with yourself and with the nursing profession and you believe that a change in both is essential for progress, give serious consideration then to the following question: Are you willing to sacrifice what you are at the moment for what you can become? (Powell, 1969). If you are committed to self-improvement, professional growth, and the value of assertiveness in helping you and the nursing profession advance, you will make the decision to be an assertive nurse and to help other nurses develop assertive skills.

References

Bloom, Lynn, Karen Coburn, and Joan Pearlman. *The New Assertive Woman.* New York: Dell, 1975.

Drucker, Peter. *Management: Tasks, Responsibilities, Practices.* New York: Harper & Row, 1973.

Gelatt, H. B., Barbara Varenhorst, and Richard Carey. *Deciding.* New York: College Entrance Examination Board, 1972.

Gelatt, H. B., Barbara Varenhorst, Richard Carey, and Gordon Miller. *Decisions and Outcomes.* New York: College Entrance Examination Board, 1973.

Hamacheck, D. E. *Encounters with the Self.* New York: Holt, Rinehart & Winston, 1971.

Hennig, Margaret, and Ann Jardim. *The Managerial Woman.* New York: Simon & Schuster, 1976.

Johnson, David W. *Reaching Out.* Englewood Cliffs, N.J.: Prentice-Hall, 1972.

Johnson, Suzanne Hall. *Assertiveness in Nursing.* Lakewood, Colo.: Author, 1980.

Kelly, Lucie Young. The Good New Nurse Network. *Nursing Outlook* 26 (1978):71.

O'Neill, Nena, and George O'Neill. *Shifting Gears.* New York: Avon Books, 1975.

Pardue, Stephanie Farley. Assertiveness for Nurses. *Supervisor Nurse* 11 (1980):47–50.

Powell, John. *Why Am I Afraid to Tell You Who I Am?* Niles, Ill.: Argus

Communications, 1969.

Raths, Louis E., Merrill Harmin, and Sidney B. Simon. *Values and Teaching.* Columbus, Ohio: Charles E. Merrill Books, 1966.

Schuller, Robert. The Theology of Self-Esteem. *Saturday Evening Post* (May–June 1980): 42–44ff.

Simon, Sidney, and Howard Kirschenbaum. *Values Clarification: A Handbook of Practical Strategies for Teachers and Students.* New York: Hart, 1972.

Stevens, Barbara J. *The Nurse as Executive.* Wakefield, Mass.: Nursing Resources, 1980.

Uustal, Diane. *Values and Ethics: Considerations in Nursing Practice.* Amherst, Mass.: Author, 1978.

Viscott, David. *Risking.* New York: Simon & Schuster, 1977.

3
Individual Rights

As Americans, individual rights are a strong part of our heritage. In fact, our country was founded on the premise that all individuals were created equal and therefore have certain inalienable rights. This chapter addresses our personal rights: those privileges belonging to individuals as they engage in the process of interacting with others in daily activities and encounters.

Women in general—and nurses, more specifically—usually do not think in terms of having personal rights. Traditionally, nurses have not asserted their rights, nor have they been encouraged to do so by faculty or administration, possibly because conflict can arise whenever personal rights are asserted. An organization may seem to run more smoothly if nurses allow their rights to be ignored. For this reason, nurses have been taught that a key part of their organizational role is to "keep the peace," often resulting in a violation of their rights. However, under the surface of a peaceful veneer, dissatisfied, disgruntled employees can cause havoc for an organization in significant ways. For example, the sense of powerlessness that stems from nurses' rights being violated can take its toll in low morale, high turnover rates, and career dropouts. Today, many nurses are discovering that their basic human rights must be recognized and exercised.

One of the goals of assertiveness training is to help you enhance your rights and the rights of others. Refusing to stand up for your individual rights characterizes and reinforces nonassertive behavior. When a nurse allows her rights to be overlooked or blocked, she often undervalues herself, fails to attain personal and professional goals, and becomes dissatisfied with herself and her life.

Why Identify Your Rights?

Identifying a specific right inherent in a particular situation makes it easier to initiate assertive behavior. Jakubowski-Spector (1973) identifies several reasons for developing a belief system about rights in conjunction with assertiveness. First, you will feel good about yourself, even if friends or colleagues disagree with you. For instance, suppose that a colleague asks you to pass prepoured medications to her patients. You believe that such a practice is unsafe, and you know that it is against hospital policy. If you believe that you have the right to refuse the request, you can feel good about yourself and the refusal even if your colleague is not pleased with your decision. Second, identifying an inherent right makes it easier for you to withstand criticism. In this example, you can handle competently whatever sarcastic remarks may come from your colleague if you are confident of your right to refuse to pass medications poured by someone else. The colleague may tease you about being too conservative, but that criticism can be handled assertively when you are comfortable with your behavior (see Chapter 5).

Third, by recognizing that a personal right has been violated, you can counteract any irrational guilt that may accompany your assertion. For instance, after returning home, you may feel guilty about your refusal to pass a co-worker's medications because you think that it may have contributed to her having to work overtime. But your refusal was honest and justified. Another assertive way of combating irrational guilt would be to offer to help your co-worker in another way. Of course, then it would be her decision whether to accept your alternative offer.

Finally, it is easier to refuse the same request a second time when you believe that you have the right to do so. Once you have refused to pass someone's prepoured medications, for example, it is easier to say honestly the second time, "I can see that you are busy, but I have made it a practice not to pass prepoured meds. What else can I do to help?"

What Are Your Rights?

Obviously, an individual must recognize what his rights are if he is to be able to make decisions about acting on those rights. Consequently, this section examines different kinds of rights, especially as they apply to nurses. Specifically, the discussions deal with the Bill of Assertive Rights, various other personal rights, sexual rights, and specific nursing rights.

Bill of Assertive Rights

If you are uncertain about what specific rights you have, you may find the following identification helpful. These rights, identified by Smith (1975), are representative of the basic rights of all people. Our discussion of them provides adaptations to nursing as appropriate. Whether you agree totally or in part with the explanations given, the material should stimulate some thoughts about your personal rights.

1. *You have the right to judge your own behavior, thoughts, and emotions, and to take responsibility for their initiation and consequences upon yourself.*

As discussed in Chapter 2, each of us has a personal set of values which influences how we think and behave. Because our values differ, our responses to situations vary. For example, assume that a problem has developed at your place of employment regarding on-call procedures, with top and middle management disagreeing about what should be done. Each person in the middle management group may approach the problem differently, depending on her values. Some may want to discuss the matter personally with their immediate supervisors; some may want to send a group letter stating the problem and suggesting solutions; some may want to request a special meeting to discuss the issue. Each person has the right to choose her approach, to judge that approach, and to be responsible for the consequences. If a requested meeting becomes destructive or a group letter is ignored, the initiators must deal with the outcomes. Being assertive means owning up to the results of your actions, whether they are positive or negative.

2. *You have the right to offer no reasons or excuses for justifying your behavior.*

Most of us have adopted the societal expectation that we must always give reasons for our behavior. Although you may feel comfortable doing so, you do not have to give reasons or excuses for your behavior. Often we feel we must say *something* and, because we think that an open reply might hurt, we give a dishonest reason or one that avoids accepting responsibility for having made the decision. Assertive behavior, however, is honest and responsible. If a friend invites you to a cocktail party at her home and you have definite reasons for not wanting to attend, you do not have to give a reason, especially if you prefer not to share the rationale for your decision. You can refuse the request assertively and enhance your rights by saying something like this:

EMPATHIC COMPONENT	"I appreciate your invitation.
DESCRIPTION OF SITUATION	But I won't be making it to the party on Saturday."

This kind of response includes the empathic component and describes the situation. An alternative follow-up comment would be something like:

ALTERNATIVE	"Perhaps the two of us can get together some evening after work."

Being assertive does not mean that you never give reasons for your behavior but rather that you have a choice. If you feel more comfortable giving a reason, that, too, is your right. But if you decide to offer an explanation, it should be done because of your concern for other people rather than because you feel controlled by them. Further, it is important to remember that if you want to accompany an assertive refusal of a request with a reason, that reason should be an honest one and not merely a fabricated excuse.

3. *You have a right to judge if you are responsible for finding solutions to other people's problems.*

Many nurses operate on the assumption that having a license to practice nursing means automatic responsibility for helping everyone solve their problems, regardless of the nurse's personal desires. We do not have to act out a "rescue fantasy" by trying to "save" everyone from their problems. Admittedly, nurses find themselves in situations in which other people—colleagues, family members, friends, and neighbors—request help in solving problems; in such cases, nurses need to recognize that they have a choice about whether to become involved. Neighborhood attorneys, pharmacists, or dentists do not feel obligated to honor comparable requests. Yet it is not uncommon to hear a nurse say that she reluctantly helped a friend or neighbor because she is a nurse.

One basic question to ask yourself is "Whose problem is it?" Is it your problem that a friend finds it inconvenient to take her child to the physician for weekly allergy shots? You do not have to give the child injections simply because you are a nurse. In such a case, it is the parents' responsibility to arrange for the child's health care. Or perhaps you have a hospitalized relative and, because you are a nurse, your family is pressuring you to discuss the case with the attending physician. Is it your responsibility to be the liaison between the physician and the immediate family? You may decide to help another family member to ask appropriate questions, but you do not have to intercede automatically.

All too frequently nurses confuse the roles of patient advocate and caretaker. In some instances, nurses have a responsibility to assist a patient through a problem-solving process or to provide him with necessary information to make a decision, but it is not always the nurse's responsibility to make the decision or to solve the patient's problem. Interestingly, finding solutions to other people's problems can be indicative of aggressive behavior (to dominate another) or passive behavior (to be manipulated by others).

One patient's daughter explained how an assertive hospice nurse helped the patient and her family to "regain their dignity" by helping them recognize their rights and determine how the patient would spend her final days. Prior to this nurse's intervention, the patient and her family had been expending large amounts of energy dealing with feelings of anxiety and anger resulting from a lack of control over the patient's care. Once the hospice nurse assisted them in establishing control without alienating the health care professionals, the family had more energy to work on their problems of where and how the patient was to die.

4. *You have the right to change your mind.*

In spite of the stereotype that promotes changing one's mind as a female characteristic, the privilege of changing one's mind is a personal right of both sexes. Too often we assume that we must live with our decisions indefinitely. On the contrary, being assertive and in control of your own life means that you may choose to change your mind about a situation.

For example, as a nurse manager, you may have agreed to assume management responsibility for a research unit. Six months later, you may decide that you are less interested in research than you originally thought. You have the right to tell your boss that you have changed your mind and prefer a different assignment. Being assertive does not guarantee that you will get what you want (in this case, a transfer), but you probably will feel better about being honest and maintaining your integrity instead of being frustrated with poor job performance or your reluctance to admit that you changed your mind. (Perhaps if you had been more assertive initially and arranged for a trial period, the situation could have been altered more easily.)

5. *You have the right to be independent of the goodwill of others.*

How many times do you find yourself saying, "I didn't want to do it, but what could I do? She's been so good to me!" Accepting material things or services from other people, especially when you do not want them, can put you in a position of feeling obligated. In other words, not asserting your right to be independent of the goodwill of others can foster feelings of dependency and lack of control.

Two class participants came to our assertiveness course seeking help in setting limits on the gift-giving practices of an extremely generous boss. For years, the boss had been buying her two subordinates gifts each time she went out of town. She also bought them extravagant presents on holidays and birthdays. Not only were the subordinates having trouble refusing the gifts but, as would be expected, they were also experiencing difficulty saying no to her in other areas. By using assertive skills, these two women were able to acknowledge her generosity but set definite limits on the frequency and type of gift giving. Interestingly enough, they reported that their boss actually seemed relieved when they initiated a discussion of the problem. Once they took more control of what they accepted from their boss, these nurses were able to set limits more effectively in other areas as well.

Other class participants have asked for help in being assertive with generous parents. One young couple visited their parents on weekends and found that every time they were ready to return home, the parents had a package for them, usually containing an overabundance of food or other items which the couple could not use. Afraid of hurting their parents' feelings and thinking that goodwill always should be accepted gratefully, the couple continued to carry the goods home, only to have them spoil or be given to a neighbor. Within a short period of time, the couple felt powerless in the situation. Recognizing that being assertive with loved ones is a high-risk situation, the couple gave considerable thought to arriving at a comfortable compromise. They acknowledged their appreciation for the kindness extended but decided to accept gifts only within reason. In class, they rehearsed their responses, and the next time they were presented with an overabundance of food, they responded as follows:

EMPATHIC COMPONENT   "We really appreciate your generosity.

DESCRIPTION OF   But Mary and I could never eat
SITUATION   that much corn.

EXPECTATIONS   We would love one dozen.

ALTERNATIVE   And we'll leave some for you to
                          share with others who would
                          appreciate it also."

6. *You have the right to be illogical in making decisions.*

Being "illogical" has an overall negative connotation and is, unfortunately, considered a female trait. Yet acting illogically can reflect a positive decision not to be restricted to rigid, so-called logical behavior.

One area outside the scientific, "logical" realm is that of perceptiveness of others. Women and nurses generally have a profound sensitivity to the feelings of others, an asset which is recognized (if only subtly) by other health professionals. For example, physicians frequently rely on nurses to determine the essence of a patient's condition when the scientific data do not adequately explain the presenting symptoms.

Early in nursing history, nurses were guided in their practice by intuition. As nurses increasingly began to use the scientific approach, they stopped trusting natural perceptiveness and began to rely more heavily on logical conclusions. While this certainly is desirable, nurses also need to recognize their right to trust their feelings and to make decisions accordingly.

For example, as a nurse manager, you may be interviewing applicants for a position in a specialized unit. You have narrowed your selection to two applicants; one has a few more years of experience than the other and logically would be the choice for the position outlined in the job description. During the interviews, you have the feeling that the other applicant could deal with the subtleties of the position more effectively, and you offer her the job. Assertive nurses have confidence in their ability to make judgments and are not afraid to make a mistake; they feel comfortable with taking risks.

7. *You have the right to make mistakes—and to be responsible for them.*

For the most part, nurses find it very difficult to acknowledge the right to make mistakes, perhaps because of reminders in school and work situations that stress the potential seriousness of making an error in dealing with patients. The graveness of making an error is not confined primarily to the clinical area but is emphasized in all aspects of nursing. At times, nurses work in critical areas, and it is possible that an error could cost a human life. Considering, though, the many nurses who make numerous decisions daily in a variety of work settings, the frequency of life-and-death decisions may be stressed disproportionately. A certain percentage of error is to be expected. If you never make a mistake, probably you are not making enough decisions.

Hand-in-hand with the right to make a mistake is the responsibility to be accountable for the consequences. For example, suppose as a head nurse you make an error in planning a vacation schedule. You schedule two nurses' vacations at the same time, short-staffing the unit. When you discover the error and approach them with your problem, they both respond that they have firm vacation plans. You had the right to make a mistake, but you also have the responsibility to deal with the consequences. Whatever plan of action you choose, finding the solution is your responsibility.

8. *You have the right to say "I don't care."*

Given our social and educational history, the right to be unconcerned is difficult for many nurses to accept. In fact, most people who enter the nursing profession have an interest in caring for others in some way. Does a nurse have the right to say "I don't care?" Is not "caring" the very essence of nursing? While caring is an integral part of nursing, it is unrealistic to expect nurses to have an emotional investment in every patient.

Norris (1973) questions how a nurse can possibly show concern, empathy, and sensitivity for many patients at the same time, as numerous work settings seem to demand. She feels the "supernurse" expectation of being all things to all people is unrealistic.

Sometimes overwhelming expectations are established by employers. As health care delivery becomes a bigger business and providers compete for patients, public relations campaigns sell the notion that the health care provider can solve all consumers' problems or meet all consumers' needs. This unrealistic expectation usually filters down to nurses, with the result that an important concept is forgotten: that while employers rightfully expect nurses to provide nursing services and while patients have the right to expect safe nursing practices, nurses have the right not to punish themselves for not "caring" about every patient all the time.

If you find, for instance, that a personality clash is seriously affecting the quality of care you are providing for a patient, be honest and assertively request a change in assignment. You do not need to announce your feelings to the patient, but you do need to be honest with yourself. Many nurses have made progress in admitting the difficulties of caring for demanding, long-term patients, as evidenced by the frequent initiation of patient conferences that include the consultation of a mental health professional to assist the nursing staff in recognizing and dealing with their personal feelings about patients, while ensuring that those patients receive quality nursing care.

9. *You have the right to say "I don't know" or "I don't understand."*

Health care delivery has become a very complex operation. Specialization and rapidly changing technology have made the maintenance of current skills a major challenge to health care professionals. Yet many nurses, especially those in middle and top management positions, feel that they should have all the answers. On the contrary, you have the right to admit your lack of information and to ask questions when you do not know or understand something. You cannot expect to have all the answers all the time.

Although in the past nurses have been taught not to question or challenge (Ehrenreich and English, 1973), nurses can promote quality patient care and actively influence developments in the health care system by learning to ask questions appropriately and assertively.

Other Personal Rights

Closely related to the Bill of Assertive Rights just outlined are certain other personal rights. These have been compiled by Baer (1976)—"The Seven Basic Inalienable Rights of Women"; and by Bloom, Coburn, and Pearlman (1975)—"Everywoman's Bill of Rights." They include the rights to privacy, to be taken seriously and treated with respect, to express feelings and opinions, to receive equal pay for equal work, and to make realistic requests of subordinates and superiors. Each of these rights is covered briefly in the following sections.

1. *You have the right to privacy.*

The right to privacy is often overlooked by nurses, who seldom make known their needs in this area. As an example, for years nurses have been content to take their breaks (if they take breaks) in a kitchen or restroom. Yet it is important for nurses to have a quiet, private place for completing the ever-increasing amount of paper work, for counseling employees, for planning patient care, and for taking scheduled, deserved breaks from their work. Medical libraries and conference rooms often remain empty while nurses conduct performance appraisals in a linen room! By asserting the right to privacy, nurses can work more efficiently and more comfortably as well.

2. *You have the right to be taken seriously and to be treated with respect.*

The right to be taken seriously often accompanies the right to respect and may involve issues as subtle as how you are addressed. A nurse working evenings in an emergency room found that one of the new medical residents with whom she worked referred to her as "the girl." He stated to patients that "the girl will be in to ask you some questions" or "the girl will prepare you for the procedures." At the end of one evening, the nurse approached the physician in private and asked in a tactful manner that he refer to her as "the nurse," "Mrs. Smith," or even "Kathy"—but not as "the girl." His face became flushed and he stammered out of the room.

The next day the nurse was called to see the director of nursing, who could not understand why the nurse objected to being called "the girl." The nurse explained that she had the right to respect from a co-worker and disliked the term "girl." After a lengthy discussion, the director still argued that it was "only a word." In exasperation, the nurse responded, "I feel differently. If it's only a word, then from now on when the physician is ready to see patients, I will tell them that 'the boy' will take care of them." The absurdity of calling a physician "boy" finally illustrated to the director how the nurse felt, and she was able to support the nurse's right to be addressed in a respectful manner. Asserting your individual rights also can reap benefits for others. In the future, the physician just described probably will be sensitive to how he addresses other nurses as well.

3. *You have the right to express your feelings and opinions.*

While the expression of feelings and opinions is desirable, there may be times when expressing them is inappropriate. It is important to recognize that you have a choice in this respect. Nurses have significant contributions to make but often do not value their own opinions or assert their right to express them.

For example, Janet, a school nurse, sat quietly during several faculty meetings while the other staff members discussed approaches to a drug problem in the junior high school. Although she had some legitimate concerns from a health standpoint about some of the policies the faculty initiated, her attitude was that if they wanted her opinion, they would ask for it. By not asserting her right to express her knowledge, feelings, and opinions, she allowed the faculty to initiate an unsafe policy with which she disagreed, while passing up the opportunity to be recognized as the health expert in the group.

4. *You have the right to receive equal pay for equal work.*

Equal pay for equal work is a right that feminists have been asserting for over a decade. Fortunately, it represents an area in which some progress has been made. Because nursing is a predominately female profession, nurses must be alert to the fact that in comparison with other professionals, especially men with similar educations and levels of responsibility, nurses are paid significantly less. Many nurses have asserted this right by filing lawsuits, claiming sexual discrimination regarding salaries. Hopefully, the precedents set by such cases will prove beneficial to other nurses.

5. *You have the right to make realistic requests of subordinates and superiors.*

If you are an employer or manager, you have the right to expect 8 hours of work from employees for 8 hours of pay. Sometimes workers lose sight of the expectations of their jobs and need to be reminded. You have the right to make requests of your subordinates. Similarly, you have the right to ask for what you want from your superiors. Too often, nurses assume that what they want is not attainable when, in fact, most issues are negotiable. While recognizing that many health care organizations have large numbers of employees and therefore must have general policies, these policies may be more flexible than realized. You might ask yourself "What do I have to lose by making a request?"—particularly if it is reasonable. It is not unusual for nurse managers to report that nurses, especially new graduates, almost never negotiate salary or fringe benefits during preemployment interviews: They accept the terms of employment as presented without asserting their right to ask for more than is offered. You have the right to ask for what you want!

Sexual Rights

A natural extension of the rights already discussed involves those associated with our sexual lives. The topic of sexual rights is mentioned here because most nurses are women, and women generally have not recognized their rights to have equal input and expectations regarding their sexual relationships. Each of the other rights previously discussed can be asserted in our sexual lives. With regard to our sexual lives, Baer (1976) identifies specific sexual rights, including the rights to understand your body, to have an orgasm, to determine the conditions of sex, to ask for specific sexual activities, to decide when and with whom to have a sexual relationship, to determine the degree of your commitment, and to be treated as a mature person.

In addition to having sexual rights in their personal lives, nurses have sexual rights in their professional lives. Nurses in assertiveness workshops have discussed how their sexual rights have been violated in work settings. On-the-job harassment can occur in any setting where males (often physicians or administrators) have power or control over female employees or students (often nurses). Sexual harassment of nurses has occurred for years as part of the myth that because nurses know so much about the human body, they are "easy prey." Young female nursing students especially have found themselves vulnerable to sexual harassment by prestigious male physicians. Reports are not uncommon that "getting locked in the crutch cupboard" with the leading orthopedic resident is expected to be viewed as a compliment rather than a problem.

When dealing with sexual harassment, two points must be considered honestly: First, has the nurse contributed to the situation? Perhaps the "seductress game" (explained in Chapter 1) began without consideration of the consequences. Once the nurse examines her own behavior, however, she has the right to change her mind and to stop playing the game. At this point, she may choose to consider the feelings of the male game player because, by her previous participation, she may have implied approval of his advances. In situations like this, being assertive involves an honest sharing of the responsibility for the circumstances.

Second, is the nurse tolerating the sexual harassment because she thinks she has no options? Will she get support for rebuffing a male staff member? Perhaps the administration considers the "old codger" harmless and close to retirement and would not take any action. Or is the offender so powerful that the administration is willing to sacrifice the job or allow the frustration of a few nurses rather than confront the harasser? Again, nursing students are especially vulnerable for they often fear dismissal if they bring an issue out into the open. Indeed, in some situations, this may occur, so dealing assertively with sexual harassment may involve risk. As noted in Chapter 2, however, nurses have a choice. If a nurse chooses to be assertive in such situations, some possible approaches are as follows:

EMPATHIC COMPONENT	"I realize I have given you the impression that your sexual advances are flattering.
DESCRIPTION OF FEELINGS	But I have come to feel degraded by these overtures.
EXPECTATIONS	I'd like our relationship to be professional and mutually respectful.
POSITIVE CONSEQUENCE	I think we could work well together within those boundaries."

If you have accepted the situation for some time because you felt powerless, you might use an approach like this:

DESCRIPTION OF SITUATION AND FEELINGS	"I admit that until now I have done nothing about your sexual advances. However, I have become increasingly bothered by them.
EXPECTATIONS	I want the advances to stop,
ESCALATED CONSEQUENCE	or I will file a complaint with the administration (or the appropriate agency)."

Of course, the most successful approach is to deal with undesirable behavior as soon as it occurs:

EMPATHIC COMPONENT	"I realize you may feel that action was harmless.
DESCRIPTION OF FEELINGS	But I dislike it when people touch me like that.

| EXPECTATIONS | I'd like it to stop." |

In some instances, the empathic component may be unnecessary:

| DESCRIPTION OF FEEL-INGS | "I don't appreciate your advances. |
| EXPECTATIONS | And I'd like them to stop." |

As another alternative, you might say something like this:

| DESCRIPTION OF SITUATION | "I'm willing to overlook that advance, |
| EXPECTATIONS | if it never happens again." |

It is helpful to prepare in advance for the possible reactions to such assertions. Contrary to popular belief, sexual harassment can be dealt with assertively without hurting the other person or degrading the nurse if good judgment is used in the choice of words and the manner in which they are conveyed.

Specific Nursing Rights

While personal rights generally are applicable to individuals' professional lives, some additional rights relate specifically to nurses. Herman (1978, p. 27) outlines several of these rights, including the nurse's right to be an equal member of the health care team.

1. *You have the right to be treated as an equal member of the health care team.*

Nurses have not been considered equal to other health professionals, partially because of archaic sexist attitudes that still prevail. Nurses are working very hard to clarify that they are not appendages of the medical profession but rather constitute a distinct and separate group of professionals providing a different but equally important service to the health care consumer. In order for true equality to occur, nursing must continue its efforts to upgrade the academic credentials of its members. While male-dominated groups such as physicians and hospital administrators continue to block these efforts, persistence will greatly influence nursing's ability to assert its right to equal status.

Sometimes the rights of an individual nurse may be infringed upon because the nursing profession in general is not respected within an organization. For example, one Ph.D. nurse reported asserting her rights with a male colleague with whom she was to collaborate on a research project. On several occasions, the colleague was quite late for their meetings, which were to be held in his office. The nurse felt that by constantly keeping her waiting, ho was indicating that he saw her time as less valuable than his. She identified her right to the same promptness that he gave to his physician colleagues. One day, after waiting 45 minutes for him, she left the following assertive message:

EMPATHIC COMPONENT	"I understand that all of us have hectic schedules.
DESCRIPTION OF FEELINGS	But I feel your consistent lateness for our mutually set meetings indicates that you feel your time is more valuable than mine.
EXPECTATIONS AND CONSEQUENCES	I will be available to meet with you again, but in my office where my time can be utilized constructively."

The assertion was successful; thereafter, her colleague was on time for their meetings. This particular nurse felt that the colleague's original behavior was primarily the result of his perception of the importance of nurses' work. Other nurses with whom he worked had always been available at his convenience, and he had not taken their work seriously. In this situation, the nurse had some power because her employer was a potential funding source for the project. One wonders if the colleague would have responded so favorably to her assertion if she had not controlled the money.

2. *You have the right to do health teaching.*

Many nurses think it is "nice" that they are permitted to do health teaching. It is time for nurses to realize that they have not only the right but also the responsibility to provide health teaching to patients. As a matter of fact, health teaching is a recognized aspect of nursing care incorporated into many state nurse practice acts. Ironically, some institutions still require nurses to obtain a written order from a physician before providing a patient with health teaching. Thus, asserting your right to do health teaching without an order in these institutions may present a high-risk situation, but such assertiveness is critical to the issue of who controls nursing.

3. *You have the right to make decisions regarding nursing or health care.*

The right to make decisions about nursing or health care is vague to most nurses who have not clearly defined for themselves what aspects of health care are unique to nursing and can thus be decided only by nurses. It may sound shocking to some to hear about nurses defining nursing for themselves, but no one can describe better what a nurse does than an individual nurse or a collective nursing organization. Through the licensing process, the public has given nurses the right to define their own profession and the responsibility to practice it safely.

Nurses need to assert this right, as physicians do. Kelly (1978) points out that when physicians are employed by hospitals, they conform to administrative hospital rules and regulations as employees, but they never permit hospital administration to dictate medical practice. In this way, physicians have protected their right to control their profession. Similarly, nurses must control nursing.

One way for nurses to maintain control of nursing is to make decisions regarding nursing. In order to achieve this goal, a nurse needs to be clear regarding her areas of authority and responsibility. For example, a nursing administrator found it necessary to hire a new head nurse for an ambulatory care unit. When the medical director indicated that he would choose the person, the nursing administrator asserted her right to make the selection. Tactfully, she told the physician that she would appreciate his advice on qualities he had found beneficial for the person in that position to possess; however, because this position was included in her budget and because the new employee would report to her, she would do the hiring. Discussing qualities or criteria with the physician was a compromise and was more objective than discussing specific applicants. When asserting a right that has previously been deferred or negotiated, it is helpful to deal in concrete terms rather than abstractions.

In other settings, nurses are often the individuals responsible for day-to-day health issues; consequently, they have the right to make decisions regarding health. This area should be defined clearly when considering a position, especially if a nurse reports to a nonnurse. For example, in a school setting, it is usually the nurse who decides whether a student is ill enough to be sent home—not the principal, who does not have the expertise to make such a decision. When nurses assert their right to control their own practice, they are acting as true professionals.

4. *You have the right to a reasonable work load.*

Frequently nurses overextend themselves and compromise on patient care issues to the extent that they give administration the impression that they can always "make do." Because nurses almost never refuse to care for their assigned patients, they often put themselves in unsafe practice situations. In some cases, this is how nursing unions began. Right or wrong, some nurses view unionization as the only way to reduce their overloads. However, even with a contract, an individual nurse must assert her rights when necessary.

For example, one class participant practiced in a small rural hospital where the nurses worked under contract. Dorothy worked the night shift where she was one of two registered nurses assigned to cover the emergency room. Frequently she found that because of call-offs, she was the only registered nurse on duty. Working on those evenings with a skeleton staff, Dorothy worried that several concurrent emergency admissions might place her in a compromising position. Although she had outlined to her supervisor on several occasions why the staffing arrangement was unsafe and, in fact, in violation of the negotiated contract, the short-staffing problem continued. After analyzing the situation from an assertive perspective and after identifying her rights and informing her supervisor, Dorothy set limits on her work responsibility and eventually filed a grievance about the staffing problem.

Your Role in Patients' Rights

Assertive people enhance their own rights while acknowledging and supporting the rights of others. Along this line, assertive nurses can play an important role in supporting and protecting patients' rights. Because health care delivery has become extremely complex, patients are sometimes lost in the shuffle. In light of these circumstances, nurses can perform a valuable function as patient advocates.

In an attempt to return patients to their appropriate pivotal position, the American Hospital Association has published a Patient Bill of Rights, which gives patients a reference point and health care professionals a standard document from which to operate. Because patients are vulnerable and dependent on health care providers, their rights must be identified and protected. Unfortunately, patients are often afraid to exercise their rights for fear of retaliation, resulting in a frustrating or painful situation for a dependent, ill person. Frequently patients have justified complaints about their care but fear that reporting them might bring further neglect or abuse.

Specifically, helping a patient to assert his rights can be as simple as assisting the patient to get the breakfast tray 15 minutes later to allow for an early bath or as complex as reporting physical abuse. In general, nurses can help a patient to assert his rights by doing the following:

1. Educate the patient that he has both basic human rights and more specific rights as a health care consumer

2. Provide written information

3. Help the patient to evaluate the advantages and disadvantages of asserting his rights

4. Assist the patient in planning for a successful assertion

5. Promise and deliver support if the patient decides to exercise his rights

6. If required, help the patient to navigate through the complaint process

7. When necessary, assist the patient in enlisting the help of an ombudsman or consumer group

An ambulatory care nurse cited the following example of assisting patients to assert their health care rights: The nurse worked in a clinic where patients usually had to wait for hours to be seen by a physician. She had tried to change the situation but had been unsuccessful. The physicians felt that their responsibilities at the hospital were foremost and that the clinic patients, who should be grateful to be seen at all, should expect to wait. Additionally, the doctors believed that their time was more valuable than the time of the clinic patients and that clinic patients could be treated differently from private patients. One patient complained to the nurse and asked what could be done about the long waiting periods. The nurse informed him of his rights, suggested that he speak directly to the physician, and helped him to prepare an assertive complaint.

Then the nurse accompanied the patient and supported his efforts. When confronted, the physician was undaunted and responded, "I am the physician. You shouldn't question me." With the nurse's help and support, the patient organized a group of several dissatisfied patients and arranged meetings, first with the clinic director and eventually with the top administrator, to voice their complaints. When the patients still experienced no significant improvement in the promptness of their care, they contacted a local consumer rights group, which finally helped in arranging for better service. Throughout the entire process, the nurse kept her supervisor informed of her actions. Indeed, this was a high-risk situation, but the nurse was committed to her responsibility as a patient advocate.

The Relationship between Accountability, Responsibility, and Individual Rights

Assertively being in control of your life and your nursing practice implies a degree of autonomy that cannot be separated from responsible behavior and accountability for your actions. This is why both responsible actions and accountability are stressed in the discussion of rights. Passos (1973) defines responsibility simply as what one ought to do and says that accountability means being responsible for what one has done. Peplau (1971) further expands this concept by describing responsibility as a charge to do something and accountability as being answerable to someone for one's actions.

Assertive behavior is responsible, and assertive people are accountable for their forthright behavior. For example, while you have the right to make a mistake, you have an accompanying responsibility to be accountable for that error. In the earlier example of the head nurse who made a mistake in scheduling two people for vacations at the same time, the head nurse had the right to make an error in scheduling, but she was also responsible for finding a solution to the problem she had created and was accountable for the consequences of that solution. If the head nurse forced one of the two staff persons to cancel vacation plans and that person resigned over the episode, the head nurse would be accountable to her boss for the consequences of her solution. The same is true if the head nurse exceeded her budget by hiring extra staff so that both people could take their vacations. By being responsible and accountable, the head nurse may have gained increased respect from both her boss and her staff, who then might choose to emulate her behavior.

Experience has shown that nurses often avoid responsibility and accountability for their actions, even in low-risk situations.

McClure (1978) states that passivity is one reason that nurses are not accountable, as indicated by some classic examples familiar to most nurses:

- The nurse who does not want to work overtime but is unwilling to be accountable for the consequences of refusal. She refuses the request, stating that her husband "doesn't allow" her to work overtime.
- The nurse who calls off duty because she is ill. She avoids both the responsibility of the call and accountability of her actions by routinely having someone else make the phone call, implying that the other person was involved in the decision and has some control over her actions.
- The committee chairperson who resigns but never directly informs the committee members, instead allowing them to discover her resignation when she does not show up for the next meeting.
- One of two people jointly planning a program who makes a unilateral decision regarding the program and delegates a secretary to be the informant.

Passive behavior can be overcome by identifying the rights of the individuals involved and by developing assertive techniques. Responsible, assertive behavior and accompanying accountability are part of conducting oneself as a professional. Nurses are recognized as professionals and are licensed to practice separately and distinct from other health care providers. To maintain this status, nurses must continue to practice in a responsible manner. They must also become more accountable to the public for their actions. Assertive nurses accept this challenge.

You Can Enhance Your Rights and the Rights of Others

Identifying your rights is one of the first steps in learning assertive techniques. Once you have identified your rights, it is easier to enhance them. Naturally, as you begin to clarify your own rights, you will become more attuned to the rights of others, and the empathic component will follow easily. By being aware of the rights of others, you will be able to determine when it is appropriate to assert your rights and when it is not. The ability to be flexible in asserting your rights is important.

An increased awareness of others' rights leads into helping patients to assert their rights. You can serve as an assertive role model for patients by being assertive with others in the presence of patients, as well as by providing patients with information and support to speak up for themselves. In a similar fashion, when you are in a leadership or teaching position, you can enhance the rights of your staff or students by being an assertive role model and by supporting their attempts at assertive behavior. Recognize that by standing up for your own rights as a nurse, you are also indirectly enhancing the rights of all nurses.

References

Baer, Jean. *How to Be an Assertive (Not Aggressive) Woman.* New York: Signet, 1976.

Bloom, Lynn, Karen Coburn, and Joan Pearlman. *The New Assertive Woman.* New York: Dell, 1975.

Ehrenreich, Barbara, and Deirdre English. *Witches, Midwives and Nurses.* New York: Feminist Press, 1973.

Herman, Sonya. *Becoming Assertive: A Guide for Nurses.* New York: Van Nostrand, 1978.

Jakubowski-Spector, Patricia. *An Introduction to Assertiveness Training for Women.* Washington, D.C.: American Personnel and Guidance Association, 1973.

Kelly, Dorothy. Professional Accountability. *Washington State Journal of Nursing* 50 (1978):22–25.

McClure, Margaret. The Long Road to Accountability. *Nursing Outlook* 26 (1978):47–50.

Norris, Catherine. Delusions That Trap Nurses. *Nursing Outlook* 21 (1973):18–21.

Passos, Joyce. Accountability: Myth or Mandate? *Journal of Nursing Administration* (May–June 1973):17–21.

Peplau, Hildegarde. Responsibility, Authority, Evaluation and Accountability of Nursing in Patient Care. *Michigan Nurse* (July 1971):5–8, 20–23.

Smith, Manuel. *When I Say No I Feel Guilty*. New York: Dial Press, 1975.

4
Examining the Way You Communicate

A significant amount of discussion has been devoted in previous chapters to the identification and implications of the various factors influencing a nurse's decision to be assertive. Such factors are part of the planning and organizing stages which are prerequisites to implementing successful assertions, especially in those conflictual or high-risk situations requiring extensive preparation. Once the decision has been made to be assertive, sufficient attention must be given to the techniques of communicating your approach in an assertive manner. Thus, the focus of this chapter is on the implementation stage and the development of the skills necessary to execute an effective assertion. This chapter discusses considerations in communication techniques and ways to present effectively the components of the assertive response/approach introduced in Chapter 1.

What Is Effective Assertiveness?

Because assertiveness is a communication technique and because communication is a vital part of interpersonal relationships, it is necessary to examine briefly what comprises interpersonal effectiveness. According to Johnson (1972), in order to be effective interpersonally, you need to be aware of the consequences of your behavior and decide whether those consequences are synonymous with your intentions. Interpersonal effectiveness then can be defined as the degree to which the consequences of your behavior match your intentions.

Whenever you interact with another person, you create some impact, evoke some impressions, or trigger some feelings and reactions. Sometimes you create the impression you want to convey, while at other times you find people reacting to your behavior much differently than you would like. An expression of warmth, for instance, may be viewed as offending; an expression of anger may not be taken seriously. Your interpersonal effectiveness depends on your ability to communicate clearly what you want to communicate, to create the impression you wish to create, and to influence the other person in the manner you intend. If, as a result of receiving feedback on your behavior, you discover that your messages are not being received as they were intended, you can modify your approach until it produces the consequences you desire (Johnson, 1972).

Likewise, effective assertiveness is concerned with whether an individual's message is interpreted and received as it was intended. It is not unusual for a person to say one thing verbally but to relate an entirely different message nonverbally through body language. To convey your message accurately, it is necessary for both your verbal and nonverbal communication to be congruently assertive.

As a part of interpersonal effectiveness, an effective assertion communicates the sender's message in an open, honest, and direct way, stating clearly the expectation desired. "What you want" as a result of your assertion, as well as the entire message, must be conveyed to the other person in an accurate, precise manner in order to maximize its chances of being heard correctly. Although the other person may not always respond by providing you with what you want, it is important for you to state your expectation in order to enhance your own self-esteem and to help the other person become more aware of your presence by your "active," action-oriented role.

Because relationships and communication involve other people, you must be accepting and responsive to them in order to be effective interpersonally. Entire books have been written on the subject of developing the skills necessary to reach out effectively and to respond to others. However, since the main thrust of assertiveness is on the "self" rather than on the "other," the focus in this chapter is on helping you to develop skills of self-expression.

Ironically, a major portion of a nurse's education is devoted to understanding and responding to the "other" (for example, the patient, the family, the physician, auxiliary personnel, and the system). While this emphasis is important and necessary, in the past there has been an excessive focus on the nurse's responsiveness to others and not enough attention on the nurse herself. Lately, however, there has been more of an emphasis placed on meeting individual nurses' needs in order to aid in retention and recruitment of nurses and preventing "burn-out." Continued attention must be directed toward helping individual nurses to feel satisfied and rewarded if the profession is to thrive.

As individuals, nurses have a responsibility to identify, communicate, and make effective assertive statements in order to obtain what is best for their own personal and professional advancement. These assertive efforts, however, should not alienate others with whom nurses come in contact since successful working relationships are imperative for advancement. Successful working relationships include cooperation with others.

Acceptance of Others

In order to establish a climate of cooperation, we must direct some of our energies—but not necessarily to the degree that we have in the past—to understanding the needs of others and communicating our acceptance of them. Harris (1967) suggests that this goal can be accomplished best by conveying to other people the idea that "I'm O.K., you're O.K." This approach reveals a positive self-image and communicates the idea that both people in the relationship are valuable and worthwhile. Mutual acceptance, respect, and support are promoted. Making a conscious commitment to relate to others in this manner will increase your interpersonal effectiveness and, likewise, enhance your chances of being successfully assertive.

When you convey acceptance to others, they must feel that you are communicating to them "You're O.K." There are times when the communication of such acceptance will lead to a generalized feeling in the other person of being supported. There are other times when the person takes a risk in disclosing something of importance, and your ability to communicate acceptance is essential for the development of trust and further self-disclosure in the relationship (Johnson, 1972).

In assertiveness, the first component of the assertive response/approach introduced in Chapter 1 is "I understand/I hear you," which can convey acceptance of the other person. It attempts to communicate empathy and understanding of the other person's position. However, it is not sufficient merely to say the isolated words "I understand" without listening with understanding and expressing warmth and caring. In order to convey acceptance of the other person effectively, both of these characteristics need to be present.

By listening to what the other person has to say, you come to understand the issue from his perspective. Unless you understand what is said, you cannot respond in an accepting way: It is impossible to accept what you do not know or understand. Listening with understanding conveys to the other person that you know what he is trying to communicate and that you sincerely want to understand him. A sincere desire to understand the other person usually is perceived as a sign of caring and a willingness to take seriously the other person's feelings and ideas. Consequently, self-disclosure continues and mutual trust develops. Further, communicating your understanding in a warm, caring way will help build in the other person a feeling that you accept him as a person. There is almost universal recognition that a degree of warmth in interpersonal relationships is absolutely essential for psychological growth. Without the communication of positive reward, you cannot communicate acceptance to another person (Johnson, 1972).

Many nurses have a natural tendency to convey acceptance of others through their warmth and caring. This characteristic is an admirable quality and one which nurses need to recognize as a positive attribute. A particular nurse who worked in the emergency room of a large, metropolitan hospital perceptively intervened on behalf of a patient's family when one night after the resident on call pronounced a given patient dead and told her that he would speak to the family by phone from his room, the nurse stated that she felt it would be more comforting for the family to speak with him in person. Recognizing the difficulty the resident had in facing the family directly, the nurse offered to accompany him and made some supportive comments to both the physician and the family.

This nurse recognized the importance of warmth and caring in communicating acceptance of family members as well as co-workers. Such concern does not imply that one must unconditionally approve of everything another person does. In fact, approval of behavior is quite different from accepting someone as a person. One can disapprove of behavior while still communicating acceptance of the person as a human being. For instance, when a co-worker's behavior warrants criticism, it can be administered in a warm, positive, constructive way without communicating rejection of the person. Although details of giving criticism assertively are discussed in Chapter 5, the following example illustrates a nurse's confrontation with a co-worker regarding assertive criticism while communicating acceptance of the colleague as a person.

When a new instructor named Beverly joined the faculty of a school of nursing, Lynn, a co-worker, was asked by the department chairperson to help with the orientation. Initially, Beverly seemed eager for Lynn's help and guidance. And Lynn felt a responsibility to help orient Beverly so that she would feel comfortable and make the necessary adjustment to become a capable, functioning member of the department. Lynn spent time sharing her knowledge verbally in addition to giving Beverly written materials to review. Lynn thought Beverly was accepting of her help but later learned from another co-worker that Beverly had ridiculed her attempts by saying that she gave her assignments and treated her like a student.

Lynn felt hurt that Beverly would interpret her assistance that way and wished that if her approach had been offensive, Beverly would have told her directly rather than talking "behind her back." Realizing the importance of their continued relationship, Lynn recognized the need to communicate warmth and caring to Beverly as a person while continuing to let her know in an open, honest, and direct way how she felt. Lynn also intended to listen with understanding to Beverly's response to her assertion because it could provide her with helpful feedback about her own behavior and could have implications for their future interactions. Consequently, Lynn proceeded to approach Beverly about the subject in this way:

DESCRIPTION OF FEEL- INGS AND SITUATION	"I'm aware that you've been feeling like a student of mine instead of a colleague. I feel badly about that since my intention was to be helpful as a co-worker by providing you with information to make your orientation to the job and the department easier.
EMPATHIC COMPONENT (ASKING FOR FURTHER CLARIFICATION AND FEEDBACK)	I realize there must have been something about my manner that precipitated your reaction, and I'd like to know more about that . . .
EXPECTATIONS	I was really surprised and hurt to learn about your reaction from someone else. I would have preferred to hear it directly from you; then we could have discussed it.
POSITIVE CONSEQUENCE	In the future, I'd appreciate your letting me know when I offend you. That way we can have a more effective working relationship."

Although this assertion conveyed Lynn's disapproval of Beverly's indirect communication via a third party, it indicated a willingness to accept constructive feedback and to evaluate and alter her own behavior in order to attain a mutually satisfying working relationship. Also, it fostered open, honest, and direct communication for the future by indicating the value of Beverly's perception of the relationship. By telling Beverly that she wanted to be informed directly of her dissatisfaction, Lynn opened the door to receiving direct feedback on her own behavior. Her ability to accept such criticism, if and when it is given, will influence the amount of trust her colleague develops in her. In other words, Lynn's future actions should support her verbal invitation for openness and honesty. This step is crucial in developing authenticity in a relationship.

Effective assertiveness is not only an expression of your perceptions and desires, but it also promotes a comparable sharing on the part of the other person. While it is certainly possible for the other person to communicate how and what he wants regardless of the quality of the relationship, in meaningful relationships the other person is much more inclined to self-disclose if he feels a sense of trust, safety, and closeness. You can foster these characteristics by conveying acceptance of him as a person.

Communicating Authentically

Because assertiveness means being honest with yourself as well as with other people, it is important to convey acceptance through listening with understanding and expressing warmth and caring only when you truly want to do so. The empathic component of the assertive response/approach should not be used automatically without feeling; instead, it should be used only when you really want to convey to the other person a sincere understanding of his position.

If you are not genuinely concerned about someone else, you should not act as though you are. If you do not feel like listening, do not pretend that you do. Most of the time, the other person will be able to detect your real feelings anyhow. Besides, your chances of gaining that person's respect will increase if you state your position honestly rather than pretending to be interested when you are not.

In conversations, you can take an active, influencing role instead of passively listening, if you so choose. During the course of a discussion, you can alter its direction actively by the comments you make or the questions you ask. If a situation is becoming boring or too time consuming, you can excuse yourself tactfully. For example, in a work situation with a verbal co-worker, it may be appropriate to say something like, "I know that you have a lot to talk about and you need someone to listen to what you have to say. Right now, though, I'm having a hard time doing that because of other things I know must be done." If you want, you might add,

"We can talk more later." This last comment may set you up for the same predicament again, so it is important to decide if you want to extend the invitation and, if so, in what setting and for how long. If the other person is someone to whom you feel a sense of responsibility (for example, a patient, subordinate, student, or loved one), you may want to make a definite commitment to get together again within a specified period of time or to provide some other means of helping the person to meet his needs.

How many times do we find ourselves listening to other people when we really would rather not? Maybe it is because as nurses and women, we are fearful of rejection and, in turn, do not want to reject others. Or perhaps we are sensitive to the dilemmas of others and feel a responsibility to provide assistance. Our socialization as women and our education as nurses have taught us to soothe others, to reach out to them by providing empathy, and to be a "good" listener. These are fine attributes when used discriminately and with appropriate limits. In fact, a number of nurses identify these qualities when asked to state a personal strength or activity that they do well. Being a "good" listener is mentioned frequently. Unfortunately, it is not unusual for nurses to relate that their willingness to listen sets them up to be taken advantage of (by certain friends, neighbors, family members, or co-workers) when they do not exert control or establish limits for themselves.

A pediatric nurse in a small community hospital shared the difficulties she was having with a subordinate who followed her around from patient to patient during morning care, discussing her personal problems. The nurse did not really want to listen but initially had acted as though she were interested. As the situation progressed, she became tired of the same barrage every time the two of them worked together. Besides, she felt that her primary responsibility of providing nursing care to the patients was hampered by her intrusive co-worker. The nurse claimed that she had tried to redirect her subordinate, but the subordinate refused to "take the hint." In all probability, the nurse's passive manner had not been direct and firm enough for the subordinate to receive the message clearly. Obviously, the situation had gotten out of hand, to the point that the subordinate expected the nurse to share her "morning care" between the patients and herself.

The nurse wanted the problem to end but was fearful of hurting her subordinate. It was suggested that she establish firm limits in a kind, understanding way, while at the same time sharing responsibility for the progression of the situation. Using the components of the assertive response/approach, the nurse planned and rehearsed her assertion. She approached her subordinate one morning immediately following report and told her that she would like to have some time alone with her in the conference room before beginning their morning routine. In a warm, caring manner, she said:

EMPATHIC COMPONENT	"I realize you like to talk with me about your personal life when we work together, and I know I've had a part in encouraging you to do that.
DESCRIPTION OF FEELINGS AND SITUATION	I've been thinking about it, though, and I feel that our time on duty needs to be spent primarily with patients doing work-related tasks.
EXPECTATIONS	I would be willing to spend either a morning or afternoon coffee break with you, but during patient care time each of us should do our own jobs. That doesn't mean we can't work together or be in the same room, but our attention needs to be on patient care.
POSITIVE CONSEQUENCE	By doing that, hopefully we will do a better job, which is what we're getting paid for."

The nurse felt very pleased with herself after executing the assertion and was relieved that the burden of an "extra patient" had been alleviated. She still felt an obligation to spend time with her subordinate during coffee breaks, but she was satisfied that limits had been established and was confident that the content of the conversations gradually would change to other topics.

As evident in this illustration, nurses often allow themselves to become victims of other people's conversations because they feel it is polite or because they do not know how to set limits and take control of their own behavior. While there may be merit to listening in that one can benefit from integrating the knowledge and experience of others, it is important to recognize that listening, like other skills, can be used selectively.

With the exception of certain listening components of the nurse's work, in many instances you do not have to listen if you do not want to listen. A superfluous telephone call or an unexpected interruption at an inopportune time can be terminated. A co-worker's abusive language does not have to be tolerated: You can walk away. Demands made on your time which you do not sanction can be limited. Of course, if an important part of your job involves listening and you find yourself not wanting to listen, especially to patients, then perhaps you should evaluate your present situation to determine if a change may be in order.

On the other hand, when you choose to listen, the extent of your attention and your listening style are a matter of choice. Superficial listening, which most people employ, does not communicate any real acceptance of the other person. When focused purposefully and used discriminately, listening can be a valuable tool to enhance relationships and promote assertiveness. Like warmth and caring, attentive, meaningful listening should be used earnestly and sincerely.

What Is Your Listening Style?

In order to communicate your acceptance of the other person through the use of the empathic component of the assertive response/approach, it is necessary to listen to what he has to say. Listening also sets the climate for an open, honest, reciprocal discussion. Consequently, a portion of this chapter is devoted to helping you evaluate your listening style and develop more effective listening skills.

Most individuals use a variety of listening styles depending upon who else is involved and their purpose for listening. Seven listening styles have been identified as those which people use in response to others' communicated messages (Pearlman, Coburn, Guest, and May, 1975). Some styles have the potential of being positive and helpful if used appropriately, while others are more clearly condescending and negative. As their characteristics are described, try to determine the type of listening style you use most frequently. As you become more aware of your own listening patterns, you may want to make some modifications in them.

The Boss

The "boss" states that things are to be done one way, according to the authority, with no room for alternatives. This style is most often found in situations where there is a defined hierarchy such as parent-child, teacher-student, or employer-employee situation.

At times, authority figures must take a definite stand and communicate firmly that their expectations are to be met. This can be done in an assertive way. However, the listening style described as "the boss" is condescending and conveys the message "If only you would have done it the way I told you, it would have worked out."

In a hospital setting, this type of response is illustrated by the supervisor who says haughtily to a flustered, short-staffed, 3:00-to-11:00 charge nurse who is explaining the difficulty she has in completing her work, "I told you last week that you needed to organize your time better." Such a remark perpetuates the frustration the nurse already feels and may intensify her anger or disrespect for the supervisor. Certainly, the nurse does not feel helped or understood.

Sarcasm

The sarcastic style of listening is composed of subtle and not-so-subtle put-downs. The sarcastic remark often takes the focus off the content of what is said and puts it uncomfortably on the person speaking or on the sarcastic remark itself. It conveys the impression that the speaker's feelings and the things she says are not very important.

For example, in response to a co-worker's expressed disenchantment regarding her inability to change the system within the nursing department, a colleague flippantly says, "Well, who do you think you are anyhow, Supernurse?" Such a curt remark leaves the person feeling dejected, with a lack of understanding and support. It may even promote animosity toward the speaker.

The Analyst

The "analyst" responds in a way that says, "I know what your problem is." The hidden message is that "you don't." Although this type of listening style has the potential of providing the other person with insight into her own behavior if used accurately and appropriately, it can also be inhibitive if used in a condescending manner or in excess because it prevents the other person from figuring things out for herself.

Consider this example: In listening to her head nurse complain about the inconsistency between shifts regarding a particular procedure, a staff nurse says, "If you weren't such a perfectionist, you wouldn't be so concerned about it." While the analysis may be accurate, chances are that in this given situation the head nurse would become defensive, especially if the remark was said sarcastically. Probably she would also look with disfavor upon the staff nurse for being offensive.

The One-Upper

In the case of the "one-upper," whatever is said is not taken seriously. The one-upper indicates that the situation is not very significant by responding with a story about herself instead. Her inclination is to "outdo" the other person.

For instance, when a nursing educator tells a colleague about the exceptional quality of her students' term papers, the colleague responds with, "You think yours are good? You should read mine! They are the best I've ever seen." Such a response undermines the speaker's intention and dissipates her enthusiasm, and it may leave her reluctant to share her accomplishments or concerns in the future with this colleague.

The Discounter

The "discounter" is similar to the one-upper in that the speaker's message is not taken seriously. But rather than trying to "outdo," the person who uses this listening style negates the other person's feelings by encouraging their denial. In an attempt to be supportive and reassuring, the discounter tells the speaker, "Cheer up!" "You'll feel better about it tomorrow" or "Don't worry about it— it will go away."

As an example, when entering a patient's room and finding him tearful and depressed, a nurse says, "C'mon, Mr. Jones. It's not that bad. Let's take a walk down the hall and visit Mr. Rupert." If the nurse is successful in convincing the patient to walk down the hall and visit with his friend, he may feel better temporarily, but his relief probably will be only short-lived. He may feel that the nurse does not understand his concerns or have the desire or ability to help him deal with them.

The Cross-Examiner

The "cross-examiner" fires a series of questions seemingly designed to obtain information. Unlike probing questions to help to clarify a situation, these inquiries are designed to "pin" something on the other person. While conclusive evidence may be a necessary intention, the results of such an approach also can be detrimental.

When a husband arrives home significantly later than scheduled, for instance, his wife may interrogate his every action: "What time did you leave the office? How long were you stuck in traffic? What stores did you go in? What did you buy? Then where did you go? What did you do there?" While appropriate questioning conveys interest and concern, such a barrage of questions intended to trap the other person can smother a relationship and perpetuate mutual feelings of distrust.

The Advice Giver

The person who "gives advice" is similar to "the boss" in that he always has the answer. The answer may be stated in the form of a platitude, such as "Children should be seen and not heard," or in the form of suggested solutions to a problem. While there are instances when providing guidance and direction to another person is necessary, the "advice giver" typically supplies them even when they are not desired. Such statements often include "shoulds" and "oughts."

For example, in response to a staff nurse's complaint about her subordinates, she is told by a co-worker, "You're just too easy with those aides. You ought to crack down on them. You should keep closer track of their time off the unit." Even though the suggested solutions may be realistic, chances are that the nurse initiating the complaint knows what "should" be done but, for a variety of reasons, has not done it. What she may want most in response to her complaint is an indication that the listener understands her plight.

Techniques of Attentive Listening

In order to respond to another person in an understanding way, you can learn to employ the techniques of attentive, or "active," listening. Attentive listening means paying careful attention to the individual who is speaking. It includes looking at the person, avoiding distractions, and sitting or standing in a relaxed and attentive position while giving short, encouraging responses. An important component of attentive listening is the use of paraphrasing: restating the person's message (that is, the ideas and feelings expressed) in your own words.

As an example, a young female patient hospitalized for diagnostic tests to rule out malignancy may share her fears and concerns with the evening nurse: "I'm really afraid to be alone. I'm afraid I'll kill myself. I don't want to, but I get so depressed. When I was at home, I was afraid to go outside for fear I would run in front of a car. I really didn't want to come in here because they might tell me I have cancer. It's horrible! My mother had it; so did my grandmother and my aunt. And when I first found this lump, I ... see ... I'm breaking out in a cold sweat just talking about it." The nurse's paraphrased response might be as follows: "You feel that you might have cancer because so many people in your family had it ... and you've been letting that fear creep into every aspect of your life. . . . "

The intent of paraphrasing is to determine whether the listener accurately comprehends the message as it was intended. Paraphrasing also can help the speaker to clarify or elaborate on his original message or deliver a new message that may be more meaningful to him. When used authentically, paraphrasing conveys that you care about what is being said and that you want to understand it. It is especially valuable at the beginning of a relationship until a level of trust is established. In addition to conveying understanding and promoting accurate communication between people, paraphrasing has the value of reducing an individual's fears about revealing himself, and it decreases his defensiveness about what he is communicating (Johnson, 1972).

Although effective responsiveness to another person is highly influenced by the intentions of the listener, the actual phrasing of the response is also important. Johnson (1972) enumerates four areas to consider when paraphrasing your response:

1. Content: The words you use to reflect back the meaning of the message should be your own rather than a repetition of the speaker's exact words. Statements that merely repeat the speaker's words do not convey understanding.

2. Depth: The degree of meaning you attach to the message should match the depth of the speaker's message. In other words, you should not respond lightly to a serious statement or seriously to a superficial one. An exception to this rule may include certain therapeutic situations.

3. Meaning: When reflecting back your perception or interpretation of the message, it is easy to add or delete meaning. Such distortion can occur because of "selective perception" wherein one hears what he wants to hear. It can
also occur by responding only to a segment of the message,
such as the last sentence. Therefore, it is advisable to paraphrase in a tentative way so that the meaning of the message can be negotiated until it is confirmed by the speaker.

4. Language: It is advisable to keep the language in the response simple in order to promote accurate communication.

To improve your skills at paraphrasing, consciously try to
paraphrase the next time you are in a discussion with someone.
Speak up for yourself only after you have first restated the ideas
and feelings of the sender accurately and to his satisfaction. Before
presenting your own point of view, try to achieve the other person's
frame of reference and to understand his thoughts and feelings
well enough that you can paraphrase them accurately. Although
this skill may sound simple, in reality it will present a challenge.
You may find that often you are sidetracked into listening to details rather than focusing on the central message, or you may be
preoccupied with formulating your own response instead of giving
your undivided attention to the speaker.

Even though active, attentive listening can promote accurate
communication, effective interpersonal relationships, and problem solving, in some instances listening alone is not sufficient. At
times, it needs to be followed up with guidance and direction or,
when appropriate, a commitment to action.

Midway through a 6-week assertiveness program, a head
nurse in the group related that she regularly used attentive listening skills with a particular staff nurse on her unit. Unfortunately,
the results were unsatisfactory, and she wanted to know where she
had gone astray. As she described it, the situation was one in which
a staff nurse complained to her about a particular aide on the unit
with whom she had been working for many consecutive evenings.
The staff nurse perceived the aide as troublesome and ineffective.
The head nurse claimed that the more empathetic she tried to be

with the subordinate by listening and "tuning in" to her concerns about the aide, the angrier and more volatile the staff nurse became. Ultimately, the staff nurse terminated the interaction in furor and disgust by saying boisterously, "I've had it! Maybe it's just time I quit." The head nurse was left feeling frustrated and puzzled because she thought that she had been using an effective technique with her employee.

In analyzing this situation, there are numerous possibilities and guidelines to consider:

1. Through direct inquiry with the staff nurse, it would be advantageous to determine the basis of her frustration. What is the underlying cause? Other factors may be contributing to her frustration besides the aide:

   a. Is the evening work load heavier than one professional nurse can handle competently?

   b. Is the staff nurse feeling inadequate about her ability to care for the numbers and kinds of patients currently on the unit?

   c. Is she feeling a lack of support and guidance from management?

   If the answers to these questions are in the affirmative, then it is the head nurse's responsibility to act in behalf of the staff nurse. She can do this either by making a verbal commitment to her subordinate that she will supply the evening shift with additional staff or by actively providing guidance in the management of the current patient census. The head nurse may choose to provide this instruction herself directly or make other arrangements via staff development, continuing education programs, or designating other staff as role models.

2. Is the staff nurse's assessment of the aide accurate? Are her expectations of the aide's performance realistic?

   a. If the head nurse does not know the answers to these questions immediately, she can inform the staff nurse that she wants a few days to collect more data and then

arrange to discuss the situation again within a specified period of time.

b. If the head nurse is already aware of the aide's capabilities and job performance, and believes that the staff
nurse's complaints are justified, she can choose either
to speak with the aide herself or to instruct the staff
nurse in ways to deal with the aide assertively. She
may want to point out to the staff nurse the merits of
taking positive action as soon as the aide's behavior
warrants it rather than building up frustration until it
culminates in an uncontrollable outburst.

The suggestion for the staff nurse to deal directly with
the aide would be especially appropriate if the head
nurse earnestly believed that the staff nurse needed to
learn more effective ways of interacting with subordinates for her own professional growth. It should not be
done, however, to "pass the buck" when the head nurse
feels reluctant to confront the aide herself.

It may even be appropriate for the head nurse to arrange a three-way meeting among herself, the staff
nurse, and the aide to try to resolve the problem. In
this approach, the head nurse should avoid "taking
sides"; rather, she should function as a mediator and
facilitator. In so doing, she could act as a role model by
teaching the staff nurse and the aide how to deal with
conflict assertively.

c. If the head nurse believes the staff nurse's complaints
about the aide are unjustified, she may want to point
out the staff nurse's unrealistic expectations of the
aide and help her to find other ways of handling the situation.

Regardless of which alternative is chosen by the head nurse,
it is important for her to follow up attentive listening with assertive
action. While attentive listening skills are important and potentially effective, in many instances they should not be considered
ends in themselves. Instead, they should be used in conjunction

with other skills, such as problem solving, guidance and direction, confrontation, and negotiation.

Assertive Verbal Communication

In addition to the relevance of attentive listening skills in assertiveness, the effective execution of an assertion is highly dependent upon one's verbal and nonverbal communication. At this point, the specifics of verbal communication are addressed; details relevant to nonverbal communication are discussed in the next section.

Words, Manner, and Timing

When implementing the components of the assertive response/approach, it is necessary to consider your choice of words, the manner in which they are stated, and the timing of the assertion. Your choice of words in and of themselves can convey passiveness, assertiveness, or aggressiveness. In response to an invitation, a comment of "Uh . . . a . . . I don't know about that place . . . the last time we went there . . . oh, you know what I mean . . ." implies that the speaker is unsure of himself and dubious about making a commitment. On the other hand, "I don't care to go," when stated with certainty and assurance, is assertive. A sarcastic statement like "You gotta be kiddin' . . . the way they treated us . . . you wouldn't catch me there!" is aggressive.

Words that convey uncertainty and avoidance are typical passive responses. The passive person is also verbally apologetic and has difficulty saying what is really meant. There is frequent loss for words, and such phrases as "I mean . . ." or "You know . . ." are used. The speech is often rambling and disconnected, indicating a difficulty in coming to the point. On the other hand, an assertive person communicates what is wanted with words that are clear and concise. Direct, objective comments made with "I" statements are spoken. Finally, an aggressive person speaks in "you" statements that tend to label or place blame on the other person. The words are accusatory, subjective, and evaluative.

Although the actual words you select are important in order to convey your message accurately, the manner in which they are stated is of even greater significance. If your tone of voice is soft and barely audible, your message probably will come across passively. A moderate-sounding voice conveys assertiveness, while a loud, boisterous tone indicates an aggressive approach.

The rate at which you speak is also an influential factor in determining whether your message is assertive, passive, or aggressive. Passive people usually speak very slowly with long pauses between words; they may even stammer. The assertive person speaks with a moderate rate, whereby each word flows evenly and regularly after the preceding one. Aggressive people tend to speak in a hurried manner with a gush of words at a rapid pace. Both the slow, deliberate, passive rate of speech and the rapidly paced, aggressive delivery can be ways of controlling conversations.

The emphasis or inflection one assigns to a phrase or series of words also has an effect on the transmission of a message. An inflection of hesitancy and uncertainty surrounds a passive approach. Assertiveness is executed in a convincing manner, while the emphasis of an aggressive style is condescending.

In addition to the importance of your method of verbal communication, consideration also should be given to the appropriateness of the timing of your assertion. Your chances of being successful will increase if you are aware of both the circumstances and the environment surrounding the situation. In determining when to initiate your assertion, pay attention to the activities in which the other person is involved, and use this information as an influencing factor in deciding when to be assertive. For example, if observations of your boss reveal that she tends to be more tolerant and accepting early in the morning than in the afternoon when the pressures of the day have accumulated, you may want to schedule an early morning appointment. Likewise, the most opportune time to approach a subordinate with a constructive criticism may not be at the end of the shift when she is in a hurry to go home. Similarly, you should determine the time of day when you function most optimally, taking advantage of the time when your skills are at their peak.

As another example, perhaps your assessment reveals that too many major changes are occurring in your institution at a given time, and you may decide to postpone presenting your idea for a new staffing pattern until some of the existing issues are resolved. Conversely, your analysis of the circumstances and environment may result in your decision to present a new approach because you believe that the best time for implementation is when the organization is in a state of change. Regardless of the specifics involved in your decision, the point to keep in mind is that the appropriate use of timing is an important factor in influencing the eventual outcome of assertions. Some additional considerations relative to timing, especially regarding expression of angry feelings, are discussed in Chapter 5.

Verbal Communication of Feelings

Verbal communication of feelings is difficult for many people. Yet the successful implementation of the second component of the assertive response/approach requires either a statement of feelings or a description of the situation. Feelings are especially difficult to express when they pertain to people in the present moment—in other words, at the time they are being experienced. Why is this so?

Johnson (1972) gives four reasons. One is that a disclosure of feelings is a risk that increases an individual's vulnerability to rejection by another person. For example, if you let another person know that you are angry with him, he may choose to avoid you. A second reason is that once your feelings are out in the open and recognized, you may feel a loss of control regarding the relationship. For instance, when expressing anger, you have no control over how the other person will react to your disclosure; he may withdraw or reciprocate with anger in an aggressive, destructive way. A third factor inhibiting the expression of feelings is that their expression often implies a demand or expectation. By stating that another person's behavior evokes angry feelings on your part, it is implied that you are requesting a behavioral change in the other person. Such demands expressed in feelings can precipitate a struggle for control between the two parties. Finally, feelings may not be expressed constructively in relationships because many people do not even recognize—much less accept—their own feelings. Without an awareness of your feelings, you cannot express them constructively.

Although the majority of nurses appear able to identify their own feelings in a given situation, some have difficulty expressing feelings. If you do, it may be easier for you to "describe the situation" when implementing the second component of the assertive response/approach. If sharing your feelings is problematic, you may want to work on developing this communication skill since sharing feelings can be a positive experience. According to Powell (1969), sharing feelings can provide you with the opportunity to know yourself and others in a new way. Furthermore, through introspection and shared feelings, you can make the necessary adjustments in your ideals and hopes for growth. As a result of this process, personal change can occur.

Describing feelings can be beneficial in that the very act of stating them to another person can contribute to your own awareness and clarity regarding your experiences. Additionally, it can provide the other person with the information necessary to respond. Sharing feelings can open up a dialogue between people. Even if the feelings are negative, they can serve as clues to what might be going wrong in a relationship and can provide the basis for a positive, constructive discussion that can lead to an improved relationship.

It is important that feelings, like ideas, are described clearly and accurately. When implementing the second component of the assertive response/approach, you can describe your feelings in any one of the following ways.

1. Identify or name the feeling: "I feel angry," "I feel frustrated," "I feel smothered," "I feel motivated," "I feel honored," "I feel satisfied."

2. Use a simile or figure of speech in which the feeling is likened to something else: "I feel as if I'm spinning my wheels," "I feel as if I'm walking a tight-rope," "I feel as if I'm on a merry-go-around," "I feel as if my hands are tied," "I feel as free as a bird."

3. State the type of action that the feeling urges you to take:

"I feel like hugging you," "I'd like to smack you," "I feel like reorganizing the whole department," "I feel like rewriting the entire manual."

If you choose to describe your feelings about another person's actions, it is wise to state them within the context of the situation and to convey that they are temporary and capable of change. It is better to communicate the message that "at this time, I am very angry with you" than to say "I dislike you now and I always will."

Such a message can be conveyed by a nursing educator who is angry with her co-worker for not delivering a message to the students as promised: "Right now, I am angry that you didn't tell the students the time and place of the test as you said you would. I've been wondering what happened to them and then found out they weren't even told!" These statements are explicit and confined to the issue at hand. In comparison, a generalization unlimited by time can be devastating—for example, "I'm so disgusted with you. I'll never trust you to do another thing."

Notice the use of "I" statements in the example. Especially when expressing feelings, it is best to use personal statements that include the words "I," "me," and "my." These personal pronouns make it clear whose feelings or ideas are being expressed. Taking responsibility for the ownership of such statements avoids ambiguity and enhances the personal quality of the communication. Personal statements also increase your chances of being understood and can help to convey your intentions of developing an authentic relationship.

Sarah, a charge nurse in an extended care facility, related how she had used assertive verbal communication with the physical therapist in her setting. He had been responsible for keeping several patient charts off the unit for an entire afternoon, which presented a problem to the nursing personnel who needed access to them. Sarah mentioned that her usual aggressive behavior would have been to attack him when he finally returned them by saying, "It's about time you're bringing those charts back! What have you been doing with them all this time? Do you think physical therapy is the only department that exists around here? Other people need to use those charts, too, you know!" Instead, because Sarah became aware of how she usually reacted in such situations, she was able to recognize her angry feelings, control them, and communicate her message not only with assertive words but also with an assertive manner:

EMPATHIC COMPONENT	"I know your department gets busy.
DESCRIPTION OF SITUATION	But the patient charts need to be available on the unit.
EXPECTATIONS	It would work well if you could limit your use of the charts to no more than an hour. If you need to keep the patients longer than that, I would appreciate your sending the charts back ahead of time.
POSITIVE CONSEQUENCES	That way, they will be available for the nurses to use as well as other departments who may want access to them."

The Relationship between Nonverbal Communication and Assertiveness

While the words individuals choose to use and the manner in which they are said are essential to convey an assertive message, nonverbal communication has even greater significance. In communicating effectively with others, it is more important to have a mastery of nonverbal communication than a fluency with words. In fact, the verbal components in a normal two-party conversation carry less than 35 percent of the social meaning of the situation, while nonverbal messages carry more than 65 percent (McCroskey, Larson, and Knapp, 1971).

The scientific study of nonverbal communication, or "body language," is called kinesics. It is a relatively new science, with initial writings published in the early 1950s. Body language concerns itself with such nonverbals as one's facial expressions, manner of dress, physique, posture, body tension, movements, and positioning as well as the degree of eye contact, touch, and spatial distance between people. All these aspects of our behavior communicate messages.

According to Fast (1970, p. 7), "We act out our state of being with non-verbal body language. We lift one eyebrow for disbelief. We rub our noses for puzzlement. We clasp our arms to isolate or protect ourselves. We shrug our shoulders for indifference, wink one eye for intimacy, tap our fingers for impatience, and slap our forehead for forgetfulness." Although much of nonverbal behavior is unconscious, it is necessary to be aware of the effect of nonverbal behavior, to learn to take more conscious control of certain aspects of it, and to understand its influence on assertiveness.

Marlene, a staff nurse in a small community hospital, related her frustrations about being the only registered nurse on evenings and being in charge of both the postpartum and the newborn nursery. Although an L.P.N. was assigned to the nursery, Marlene realistically felt an overwhelming sense of responsibility and identified the situation as an unsafe one for patient care. She expressed her concerns to Mrs. Burgess, the supervisor, a number of times, and additional staffing was promised. On the evening following the latest interchange between Marlene and her supervisor, she went on duty to find no additional help and the supervisor on vacation for the next 2 weeks. The relief supervisor, Mrs. Hines, explained that she was unaware of the long-standing problem.

Marlene reiterated her concerns to Mrs. Hines by saying:

EMPATHIC COMPONENT	"I realize that you're filling in for Mrs. Burgess, and you may not be aware of what has occurred between the two of us.
DESCRIPTION OF SITUATION	I have expressed my concerns repeatedly about being put in charge of both the postpartum unit and the newborn nursery. I cannot possibly take responsi-

bility for both areas and ensure safe patient care. Mrs. Burgess promised additional staffing for this evening. Now I find that there isn't any, she's on vacation, and I'm in the same situation as before.

EXPECTATIONS

I expect another R.N. to be on the unit within an hour to work in either of those areas. I will be responsible for only one of them.

CONSEQUENCES

If I do not get additional help, I will follow up our conversation with a memo."

Certainly, there was a risk involved in taking such a firm stand, but Marlene was so convinced of the value of her conviction that she was willing to accept whatever consequences might result. In considering Marlene's comments, they appear to be very assertive: She included empathy, a description of the situation, and a statement of expectations, and she was open and honest about the consequences. But we cannot claim that her behavior was assertive merely by examining her words. The nonverbal aspects of her approach played a significant part in how the message was transmitted. Even if verbal components are direct and appropriate, their impact can be enhanced or diminished if the nonverbals are not complementary.

The following hypothetical situations examine more closely the various nonverbal approaches Marlene could have used in communicating her message. By comparing these three approaches, you will see how body language and manner of execution can convey entirely different messages.

1. *Passive nonverbal communication*

When Marlene approaches Mrs. Hines, she is teary eyed and wringing her hands. Her shoulders are stooped; she shifts her weight

from one foot to the other and avoids looking at Mrs. Hines directly. She leans up against the hall corridor for support and, when she
begins to speak, her voice is soft and hesitant, with long pauses between her words. She looks tense and apologetic. As she states the
components just mentioned, she stammers and acts as though she
needs someone to help supply her with each word. She states the
consequences of her assertion in a questioning manner, as though
she is asking for Mrs. Hines's approval. Her concluding remarks
are followed by nervous laughter.

This nonverbal behavior would convey a double message and
indicate that while Marlene wants additional staffing and relief from
the total responsibility of two areas, she is not very serious about
either her expectations or the consequences to which she alluded.

2. *Aggressive nonverbal communication*

If Marlene spends half of the shift stewing about the situation while she madly scurries around trying to cover both the postpartum unit and the newborn nursery before finally deciding to approach Mrs. Hines, it is quite possible that she will react aggressively. By being nonassertive for an extended period of time, by
passively waiting and hoping to get some help, and by denying her
own needs and desires, the hostility and frustration Marlene has
felt for a number of evenings probably will explode. When it does,
she may say the exact same assertive words mentioned previously, but in a forceful, abrupt nonverbal way.

All of a sudden, she may slam down the charts in the nurses'
station, screaming at the aide, "I've had it! I'm going to see Mrs.
Hines!" After stalking off the unit, she might knock loudly on the
supervisor's office door and enter immediately without waiting for
a response. With a flushed face, her eyes stare and pierce. With her
feet apart and her hands on her hips, Marlene may begin shouting
at Mrs. Hines and pointing her finger in a demanding way.

Her condescending tone of voice and the rapid pace of her
words clearly would be meant to keep Mrs. Hines silent until Marlene finished. Although the content of her words might be assertive, her nonverbal message would be dominating and clearly aggressive.

3. *Assertive nonverbal communication*

In contrast to these two approaches, Marlene has the option of conveying her message in an assertive manner. At the beginning of the shift, let us assume that when she enters the unit, she learns there is no additional R.N. assigned to the shift, and Mrs. Burgess, who is unexpectedly on vacation, has been replaced by Mrs. Hines. She feels herself getting angry but is able to control her anger and use it in a constructive way. She thinks to herself, "Well, I'd better take a firm stand. This has been going on long enough!"

She asks one of the daytime R.N.s to stay a half hour overtime to cover for her while she goes to Mrs. Hines's office quickly. As she faces the door, she stands up straight and knocks firmly. When Mrs. Hines says "Come in," Marlene enters, faces her directly, and says in a relaxed way, "I want to speak with you about the situation on 4-East." Then she sits down facing Mrs. Hines, and in an assured manner with a well-modulated voice, proceeds in an open, direct way with her assertion.

She conveys caring and strength. She is at ease but does not laugh or disqualify her message in any way. She is firm in a manner that indicates her expectation of being taken seriously. Her tone of voice and her body movements reinforce her assertive words.

Physical Positioning and Environmental Surroundings

Besides personal body language, the environment in which people interact and the physical position they take in relationship to others can also communicate messages. Physical positioning and personal space between individuals are aspects of nonverbal communication that have implications for assertiveness. Positioning oneself in relationship to others according to height or spatial distance can be unconscious or purposefully used to achieve a desired result. Standing while the other person sits can convey superiority, authority, or even a time constraint. Dominance through height can be an aggressive maneuver designed to intimidate another individual when the body language conveys the idea that "I am higher and more important than you are; therefore, I am dominant." The physician who stands during a discussion with a nurse who remains seated and the nurse who stands instead of sitting or bending down alongside a prone patient are examples of dominance by height.

In addition to height positioning, the spatial distance between people is significant and can have different meanings for different groups of people. A person from one cultural background may perceive standing close to another individual as a sign of warmth, while a person from another cultural background may interpret the same distance as a sign of aggressiveness or hostility. Close body proximity is accepted as the norm for those professionals working in health care settings who perform daily direct service to patients' bodies. On the other hand, people in the business world, because of the nature of their work, are not as body oriented and have more definitive territorial boundaries.

In practice, the physical invasion of a person's territory has been found to be extremely useful in breaking down an individual's resistance. The police are well aware of this fact and take advantage of it in their interrogation of prisoners. The questioner may begin with his chair 2 or 3 feet away from the suspect, and, as the questioning proceeds, he will move in closer so that ultimately one of the subject's knees is almost between the interrogator's two knees. When an individual's territorial defenses are weakened or intruded upon, one's self-assurance tends to grow weaker (Fast, 1970).

In the work setting, the boss who is aware of this fact can strengthen his own position aggressively by intruding spatially on a subordinate. The supervisor who leans over the head nurse as she compiles a special report may contribute to the latter's feelings of uneasiness. The nursing instructor who crowds next to the student in an overbearing, hypercritical way can contribute to the student's feeling insecure. Even the parent who reprimands a child by leaning over him is compounding the relationship between them by proving and reinforcing parental dominance.

Conversely, the selection or maintenance of a seating position at a lower level or one which is more spatially distant from others can convey inferiority, passivity, or detachment. Such a position can put you at a disadvantage from the onset of an interaction.

An example of this occurred during an orientation session for new board members of a community mental health agency. A nurse from the agency, who was designated to present part of the program along with other staff members, entered the room in a sheepish manner. She walked behind the circular arrangement of chairs and began conversing informally with some of her co-workers who were already seated. She proceeded to sit down on the floor behind them, even though there were several chairs available in the circle. She remained there until she was called out of the room by a secretary requesting that she tend to a patient "in crisis." Meanwhile, other staff members were available on the crisis team who could have been paged. Interestingly, the nurse did not return to the group. One could speculate that the interruption may have been purposeful and welcomed.

As this example illustrates, the value that a nurse places on herself in terms of her own ability to contribute as an active, productive member of a group can be revealed, at least in part, by her selection of a seating position as she enters a room. Does she join others readily and situate herself in a position that reflects her assertiveness and promotes collegiality? Does she sit in leadership territory in the forefront or at the head of the table? Does she locate herself passively out of view or sit in the rear of the room off by herself in a remote area?

Where do you sit and how do you position yourself at work; in the classroom; in the nurses' station; in relationship to patients; in relationship to colleagues from other disciplines? Does your body language reflect boredom or interest? Do other people receive the message that you are concerned, or do they see you as aloof and distant? Do you communicate assertiveness, aggressiveness, or passivity through your body positioning?

You may want to be more conscious of placing yourself in an assertive position of equal height, within a comfortable spatial distance from others, and in a seating position that promotes the goals you want to accomplish in a given situation. Seating positions are sometimes indicative of one's status within a group. It is not unusual, for instance, for the leader or the person with the highest position to sit at the head of the table and for one's status to decrease as the distance from the leader increases.

The significance of seating positions and their relationship to status are evident in a particular psychiatric facility. In addition to providing patient care, this particular hospital is also oriented toward research and education. Staff seating arrangements at the weekly clinical conferences held primarily for the purpose of educating resident physicians are clearly status oriented. Seated at a front table facing the attendees is the psychiatric resident responsible for presenting the case, a staff psychiatrist, and the patient who is to be interviewed. Other participants and conference attendees sit in rows on either side of the head table. Although there are no physical markings or verbal directions regarding seating location, one needs to attend such a conference only once to learn the definite territorial boundaries that have been established by years of tradition.

The first rows on both sides of the head table are always comprised of resident physicians. The social worker and psychologist involved in the case are located nearby. The nurse who presents the patient's recent behavior may or may not be seated along with the other team members, depending on her own degree of comfort in the "presentor's" territory. More often than not, she sits behind the other professionals. The placement of the rest of the attendees is in direct proportion to the degree of status held by their respective professions in the institution, with psychologists and social workers sitting closer to the front of the room and nurses in the rear.

An assertive nurse who values her own knowledge and ability would speak out appropriately and contribute her ideas to such a conference. Assertive nursing educators would influence a change in the structure and format of the conference to provide for nursing faculty and appropriately prepared nursing students to have direct input into the presentation of the conference. While it is true that traditions are an important part of our heritage and greatly influence our current functioning, assertive nurses should not be content merely to live in them but instead must work to create them.

In addition to physical positioning and spatial distance between people, the furniture and external objects in the room also affect the communication process. Generally, round tables are conducive to informality and promote equity among group members. Rectangular tables, on the other hand, are more likely to be used in formal situations where one's status and position are of greater significance. A desk or table between individuals tends to indicate formality or status and promotes distance between people as opposed to a surrounding in which people sit in comfortable chairs with no physical barriers between them.

A nurse who is aware of spatial implications can use the external environment assertively to supplement her interpersonal dialogues with others. A particular nursing education administrator has an office that contains, in addition to her desk and desk chair, a couch, an easy chair, and a coffee table with one or two chairs around it. She communicates the formality or informality of a situation by where she sits. If a visitor comes whom she wants to treat in an informal manner, she moves from behind her desk and guides the visitor to the couch, to the easy chair, or to the coffee table. In this way, by her positioning, she assertively initiates the type of interview she will have. If it is to be formal, she remains seated behind her desk.

Physical objects between people as well as various other room furnishings such as carpeting, draperies, and style, texture, and color of the decor can contribute to the creation of either a positive or negative environment. In turn, the environment can influence the behavior of the people involved.

One nurse mentioned how the surroundings and physical position between herself and a particular male subordinate influenced a performance appraisal conference. Mrs. Meyers, a large woman, was seated behind her desk when the employee entered her office. She remained seated and directed him to an overstuffed chair alongside her desk. He sank into the chair, which put him in a significantly lower position than his boss. Immediately, he became uncomfortable and said to her in a joking manner, "What are you trying to do—make me feel small?" Mrs. Meyers was startled but pleased that the employee could verbalize his discomfort. He had helped her to become more aware of the impact of the external environment on their interactions. Subsequently, she rearranged her office furniture so that others would sit at eye level, thereby promoting more equitable and effective relationships.

When giving or receiving performance appraisals, you may want to take some assertive initiative regarding the location of the conference. Holding it in a meeting room near the unit can build in privacy and communicate the seriousness of the session. Giving employees a choice of location can communicate respect and equality. Selecting a special area of the facility to begin an important project, such as the room in which the board of directors meets, can convey to people that the task is special and their ideas highly valued.

While comfortable, pleasant external surroundings are an asset and are worth using in a positive way, they should not be used in isolation and do not take the place of effective day-to-day human interaction. Rather, they are to be employed whenever possible to enhance the communication process and contribute to the ongoing development of constructive interpersonal relationships.

The development of constructive interpersonal relationships is dependent upon effective day-to-day interaction. As emphasized at the beginning of this chapter, the core of effective daily interaction, and likewise, effective assertiveness, is when the consequences of a person's behavior accurately match his intentions—that is, when the sender's messages are received as intended. It is not unusual, however, for an individual's nonverbal communication to obstruct this process. Because nonverbal messages typically are ambiguous, the receiver may be confused about the real meaning of the message.

Nonverbal Communication of Feelings

Nonverbal behavior is used primarily to communicate feelings, likings, and preferences. Customarily, nonverbal behavior reinforces or contradicts the feelings that are communicated verbally (Johnson, 1972). Just as it is important to examine ways people can express feelings verbally, it is also important to understand how feelings are communicated nonverbally and how nonverbal expression can either impede or contribute to an effective assertion.

Feelings can be expressed nonverbally through various types of body motion. While other parts of the body certainly are used, eye contact and facial expressions are particularly revealing. Sparkling eyes and a smile indicate happiness, warmth, and pleasure. These nonverbal messages communicate friendliness, a spirit of cooperation, and acceptance. On the other hand, a frown, raised eyebrows, or rolling eyes can be indicative of disgust, disagreement, or boredom. Head nodding usually conveys agreement with the speaker, while head shaking communicates disagreement. According to Johnson (1972), there appears to be more eye contact between people who like each other than between people who dislike each other.

Because feelings are communicated more by nonverbal cues than by the words a person uses, their accurate understanding is dependent on the receiver's interpretation, which may or may not be correct. It is often difficult to know what another person really feels. A co-worker may act as though she likes you, but somehow you feel that she is being insincere. The ambiguity that can arise in the nonverbal expression of feelings is related to the fact that there are varying degrees of feelings. Furthermore, the same feeling may be communicated nonverbally in different ways by different people. For instance, anger may be expressed by a temporary sulk, a quick slam of the door, great bodily motion, or a frozen stillness that seems to last forever. When feelings are hurt, one individual may cry while another may withdraw and become aloof and distant.

In addition, any single, nonverbal cue can arise from a variety of feelings. A blush may indicate embarrassment, pleasure, or even hostility. It is understandable, then, that the receiver of a given message may be unclear about what is being communicated and, consequently, misinterpret the sender's message.

The Necessity of Congruence: Is Your Body Language in Harmony with Your Assertive Words?

In addition to the ambiguity of nonverbal messages, the fact that there are frequent contradictions between an individual's verbal and nonverbal communication contributes to the misunderstanding and misinterpretation of feelings. It is not unusual for people to say one thing and do another. A staff nurse may indicate verbally to the head nurse her willingness to work evenings on a designated date but then act antagonistic and uncooperative regarding her assigned shift. Or an instructor may tell a student that she is welcome to come to her office for additional help and then, when the student arrives, act disinterested and annoyed about the "imposition."

Everyone has at some time received or sent conflicting messages. The boss who insists that her employees get to work on time while she is habitually late, and the nursing instructor who claims she is always available to students as she continually looks at her watch and packs her briefcase hurriedly, are examples. Perhaps a co-worker may lead you to believe that she will keep confidential the information you have shared with her. Later, you discover that other employees know all about your difficulties with the boss.

Conflicting and contradictory messages are known as "mixed messages" or "double binds." They violate the basic principles of effective communication and promote anxiety and distrust among people. When receiving such conflicting messages, we tend to believe the message that we perceive to be hardest for the other person to conceal. This is often the nonverbal one. Because the nonverbal message is more powerful in communicating feelings, it is essential when executing an assertion to give particular attention to your nonverbal communication. In order for your assertion to be effective and for the other person to believe that your behavior is real and genuine, your verbal and nonverbal messages must be congruent.

Does your nonverbal behavior support your intentions to have other people take your assertions seriously? Do you speak as if you expect others to pay attention to you, or does your body language disqualify your verbal message? Is your body language so intense and overwhelming that the recipient of your message is too distracted even to focus on your assertive words? What discrepancies are there between what you say, how you feel, and how you act?

Beth, an office nurse, shared her perplexity over the ineffectiveness of her so-called assertions with her boss. She could not understand why her physician-employer criticized her periodically for leaving work on time when she had "assertively" explained to him her rationale. Beth made it clear to her boss when she accepted the position, and numerous times after that, that her role as a single parent was an important one and that she needed to leave the office promptly at 5 P.M. She worked very efficiently during the day to get her work done, sometimes even taking less than her allotted lunch time. However, occasionally appointments would be delayed or overscheduled at the request of the physician so that at quitting time, patients would still need to be seen. There was no overtime remuneration for the office personnel.

Beth had been assertive by following through persistently with her intentions to leave on time. However, her manner and body language when leaving were clearly nonassertive, especially in response to her boss's snide comments that were made under the guise of a joke. Such remarks included, "Well, there she goes, leaving us high and dry" or "What do you have under your seat—a keg of dynamite?" On closer examination, we learned that Beth's relationship with the physician was a frivolous one. Her usual response to his "jokes" about her leaving on time was to giggle sheepishly and inch her way out. She never let him know that his remarks were upsetting or that she expected to be taken seriously. Instead, her giddy behavior conveyed the opposite message and served to perpetuate his comments.

You Can Use Assertive Communication Skills

Your assertions can be successful if you learn to evaluate the outcomes of a situation, determine what is contributing to its effectiveness or lack of it, and modify your approach accordingly. Assertive communication includes the proper use of listening skills, verbal communication, and nonverbal communication. All must be in harmony—that is, be congruent with one another—in order for your assertive message to be received as you intend it to be.

Become more aware of your interactions and the way in which you present yourself in interpersonal situations. Does your behavior say "I'm not important. Don't pay attention to me"? Is it rude, cold, or inappropriate? Do you convey an air of superiority? Or are you warm, tactful, and considerate as you chart your course, state your assertive words, and attempt to do what is best for you and the nursing profession? By practicing the assertive communication skills described in this chapter, by determining to succeed, and by supplying yourself with the necessary knowledge, guidance, and support, you will be successful.

References

Fast, Julius. *Body Language.* New York: Pocket Books, 1970.
Harris, T. A. *I'm O.K.—You're O.K.* New York: Harper & Row, 1967.
Johnson, David W. *Reaching Out.* Englewood Cliffs, N.J.: Prentice-Hall, 1972.
McCroskey, J. C., C. E. Larson, and M. L. Knapp. *Introduction to Interpersonal Communication.* Englewood Cliffs, N.J.: Prentice-Hall, 1971.
Pearlman, Joan, Karen Coburn, Peggy Guest, and Cheri May. *Assertive Training for Women—A Training Manual.* St. Louis: University of Missouri, 1975.
Powell, John. *Why Am I Afraid to Tell You Who I Am?* Niles, Ill.: Argus Communications, 1969.

5
Overcoming the Inhibitors of Assertiveness

"If I assert myself and call Dr. Smith in the middle of the night to tell him about this patient's condition, he'll get angry. When he gets angry, I'll be devastated."

"If I tell the nursing assistant that he isn't doing his job well, he'll be hurt. If his feelings are hurt, it's my fault."

"It's wrong for me to refuse to work a double shift. After all, the hospital is short-staffed, and the patients need care. If I don't stay, the patients will suffer."

"One portion of the budget doesn't sound right to me, but I don't know enough about finances to give a specific criticism. If I say something, my lack of knowledge will show and the accountant will think I'm stupid."

These attitudes are examples of irrational beliefs that inhibit assertive behavior. Learning to change irrational beliefs to rational thinking can result in successful assertions.

What Are Irrational Beliefs?

Irrational beliefs focus only on the negative outcome of an assertion and distort reality (Ellis and Harper, 1974). Such beliefs may occur when a person is anxious about the outcome of a situation and is not confident of his ability to deal with the possible results. Often a person expends all his thoughts and energies on the worst possible outcome and finds himself thinking, "What will I do if . . . ?" or "I know I will fall apart when. . . . "

Irrational thoughts prevent individuals from asserting themselves and can affect their choices. Thinking about negative consequences is frightening, uses large amounts of energy, and can increase anxiety. So much energy is dissipated on the anxiety that little or no energy remains to support assertive behavior. Because irrational thinking focuses exclusively on such disastrous outcomes, the choice of whether to be assertive seems removed. Because people generally avoid unpleasant situations, it is understandable that a person is reluctant to behave assertively if a negative outcome is deemed certain.

Changing Irrational Beliefs to Rational Ones

Seven irrational beliefs and accompanying rational counterparts have been identified by Bloom, Coburn, and Pearlman (1975). By providing rational counterparts, these authors focus on reality as well as the possible positive outcomes of the assertions.

1. IRRATIONAL BELIEF — If I'm assertive, I'll hurt others.

   RATIONAL COUNTERPART — The other may or may not be hurt; he may prefer being open and direct too.

This first irrational belief is illustrated by an example from a community health setting: You and a colleague both visit a patient who has stasis leg ulcers. The care plan outlines daily soaks and dressing changes to be done by the registered nurse. You soak the leg and change the dressing each time you visit, noting that your colleague charts the same procedure during her visits. For the past few weeks, you have noticed that the healing process has slowed considerably. During one of your visits, the patient remarks that your colleague has been rushed recently and has not been soaking the leg prior to changing the dressing. You want to say something to your colleague but are sure she will be hurt. That may or may not be true. Being honest and direct does not always hurt other people's feelings. Indeed, she may know that cutting corners is a bad habit, and she may respect your concern for patient care. Further, she might appreciate hearing the comment from you directly rather than from her supervisor. Your approach to this colleague might include statements like these:

EMPATHIC COMPONENT	"I know you have been especially busy lately.
DESCRIPTION OF FEELINGS AND SITUATION	But I'm concerned about Mrs. Jones's leg ulcer. The healing process has stopped. I understand you have been omitting the soaks.
EXPECTATIONS	The soaks are part of the plan and have to be done.
POSITIVE CONSEQUENCE	If we both follow the care plan, the leg should heal completely."

Responsibility for other people's feelings often is associated irrationally with the fear of hurting others.

2. IRRATIONAL BELIEF	If my assertiveness hurts others, I'm responsible for their feelings.
RATIONAL COUNTERPART	When I'm assertive, I can let others know I still "care." My assertiveness will not "shatter" anyone. They're not that fragile. Relationships can take "ups" and "downs."

Assuming that you are the community health nurse just mentioned, you may feel responsible for your colleague's anticipated feelings. A more rational approach would be to recognize that the colleague has a "choice" regarding how she can react to the assertion. If she chooses to feel hurt, that feeling is coming from within her; in such a case, she received your message, processed it, and chose to react in an offended manner. The assertive message focuses on the behavior involved and assures that the other person is not the victim of a verbal attack.

Another area of irrational thinking centers around the idea that asking a question or making a mistake makes a person look stupid. In reality, though, it is not possible to have all the answers all the time.

3. IRRATIONAL BELIEF	I must avoid asking questions that make me look stupid.
RATIONAL COUNTER-PART	It's human to lack information or make a mistake.

For instance, suppose that recently you were asked to serve on the board of directors for a high-rise apartment building for elderly citizens. During a budget review presented by an accountant board member, you learned that an exorbitant sum of money had been appropriated for the clinic facility. You want to question that segment of the budget but are afraid there may be some fiscal principle involved and that by questioning that section, you will show your lack of knowledge about budgets. It is irrational, however, to focus only on this one possible outcome. In reality, you can discuss the concept of finances for the clinic facility without knowing all the details of the budgeting process. Besides, as a board member, you have the right to question the specifics involved in arriving at the current budget. Hence, it would be very appropriate to say something like:

DESCRIPTION OF SITUATION	"That sounds like a lot of money to be allocated for the clinic.
EXPECTATIONS	I'd like to know how you arrived at that figure."

Learning to Say No

A fourth irrational belief relates to refusing legitimate requests.

4. IRRATIONAL BELIEF — It is wrong for me to turn down legitimate requests.

RATIONAL COUNTER-PART — Legitimate requests can be refused. I can consider my needs first. I can't please everybody all the time.

Often nurses find it difficult to refuse a legitimate request regardless of their own feelings or desires. Somewhere in childhood and educational experiences, the irrational belief was instilled that you should always find the time to do something for a good cause. In other words, if someone needs you, you assume that you should forget about your own needs and rights because the other person is more important. The rational counterpart to this irrational belief is that it is permissible to consider your own needs. You do not need to please other people all the time.

For example, an assertive response to a request to work a double shift could be handled by saying:

EMPATHIC COMPONENT — "I realize you are in a bind.

DESCRIPTION OF SITUATION — But I am physically and mentally drained after an eight-hour shift.

EXPECTATIONS — I won't work a double shift and give substandard care.

OPTIONAL ALTERNATIVE — Although I'm scheduled to be off, I'd be willing to work daylight tomorrow if that would help."

Nurses often hold to the irrational belief that if they say no, the initiator of the request will be angry, upset, or disappointed. Focusing only on potential negative outcomes prevents considering that the initiator may have expected you to decline, that the initiator may be accepting or indifferent to your response, or that you may be only one of several people to whom the request was made.

The Consequences of Not Saying No

As nurses, we often find ourselves passively assuming responsibilities that are beyond our capabilities because we do not realize that we have a choice. We rationalize nonassertive behavior by saying, for example, that if we do not work as lone professionals in settings requiring three nurses on all shifts, the patients will not receive care. The reality may be that by working consistently understaffed, we are contributing to an unsafe level of care.

In this type of situation, the inability to say no may lead to inferior patient care and consumer complaints. The overworked nurse who is unable to say no often appears incompetent to the consumer because she is too busy with additional responsibilities to do the assigned job properly. Consumers who do not receive the expected level of care cannot be expected to know that a particular nurse was on duty for 14 hours; they see only the effects of the nurse not answering the call lights promptly.

The following is an illustration of setting limits assertively in order to assure safe patient care. You work the 11:00-to-7:00 shift in a critical care unit that is scheduled for three registered nurses. When you report to work, the supervisor informs you that the unit is short staffed and that you will have to work alone. You are convinced that this situation is unsafe and that it is impossible for you, as the only professional, to provide the level of care indicated. Rather than jeopardize your license and compromise your standards, you tell the supervisor assertively:

EMPATHIC COMPONENT	"I realize that you are in a dilemma with two nurses calling off.
DESCRIPTION OF SITUATION	But I cannot provide safe nursing care to the entire patient census.
EXPECTATIONS	I can be responsible for one-third of the patients, or I will be willing to work elsewhere. I will

not be responsible for the entire unit."

In addition to affecting patient care, the nurse may be affected personally by the consequences of not setting limits. When she is overworked and frustrated for an extended period, her individual or family health may suffer. Some nurses also become overextended in the interest of personal advancement. Many, because of their capabilities, are often encouraged to fulfill demanding positions of leadership and, consequently, assume excessive responsibilities. Other nurses routinely create their own stressors and crises as a way of forcing themselves into action: The nurse who has been wanting to change positions for a long time, but has never seriously explored other employment opportunities, suddenly quits her job. Or the nurse educator who has been wanting to expand her presentation but has not done so accepts a speaking engagement requiring the development of new material.

While such strategies can accomplish desired tasks, it is important to maintain a balance between creating your own crises and challenges, and establishing personal limits on what you will and will not do. Refusing to take on another demanding task when you are already stretched to capacity is being assertively responsible for your own self-management. In many different respects, nurses must learn to say no.

An essential step in saying no is to identify the types of situations in which you have the most difficulty refusing a request. Do you have a hard time refusing to buy unnecessary items from the handicapped? Refusing to go out of your way to drive someone home? Refusing to buy a raffle ticket from your boss? Identifying your specific roadblocks will help you to anticipate and plan for refusing future requests.

As you develop assertive skills, it will be helpful for you to examine the various types of people with whom you have contact—such as peers, subordinates, authority figures, loved ones, and children—in order to determine which kinds of relationships present the most difficulty to you in being assertive. Knowing, for example, that you have trouble being assertive with children, especially when they come to your door as vendors, can help you to work harder at saying no in such instances—if that is what you want to do. Realizing, on the other hand, that you are uncomfortable with authority figures, you can be alerted to your need to spend more preparation time rehearsing an assertion directed to your boss.

In addition to the fact that different situations and people can be blocks to you in terms of assertiveness, another common roadblock is guilt. Guilt is an uncomfortable feeling that individuals would prefer to avoid. However, while you may prefer being "guilt-free," that is not always possible. It is important to recognize that if you really want to, you can say no even if you feel guilty.

Guilt feelings often are the result of years of experiences that include plenty of "shoulds" and "oughts." If these expectations are evaluated honestly, though, you may conclude that refusing a request assertively does not have to end in uncomfortable feelings. Calling to mind the discussion of personal rights and overcoming inhibitors of assertiveness can result in the reduction or elimination of guilt feelings.

Consider a situation wherein a mother wants to take a class at the same time her child wants her to drive him to swimming practice. Using the components of the assertive approach, this mother might say:

EMPATHIC COMPONENT	"I understand that you want to be on the swim team.
DESCRIPTION OF SITUATION	But I am not available to drive you on Tuesday evenings for the next six weeks.
EXPECTATIONS	It will be necessary for you to make other travel arrangements.
ALTERNATIVE	Perhaps one of Joe's parents could drive you both to swimming practice, and I could drive you both to Scouts."

Another approach would be the following:

EMPATHIC COMPONENT	"I know how important the swim team is to you.
DESCRIPTION OF FEEL-INGS	But I have a right to an evening by myself.
EXPECTATIONS	It will be necessary for you to make other transportation arrangements for the next six weeks.
POSITIVE CONSEQUENCE	If you are responsible for your own transportation one day a week, I will feel better about driving you on the other days."

In this example, the mother is enhancing her own right to some private time as well as promoting independent behavior in the child. In fact, saying no often fosters an independent relationship. It is important to realize that the price you may pay for taking control of your own life is that other people may not always continue to approach you for help. If your nurturing proclivities rely heavily on people needing you, you may want to examine potential ambivalence—that is, you may want to set limits but also want to be needed.

On occasion, although you refuse a request assertively, the other person may persist, hoping that you will change your mind. After trying other approaches, eventually you may choose to escalate your assertion by saying, "I have thought about it. I have made up my mind and will not change it."

Assume that you are a single nurse-researcher involved in clinical studies with patients who have a rare endocrine disease. One of your male patients repeatedly has asked you for a date, and you consistently have turned him down in a kind but firm manner, pointing out that you prefer to keep your personal and professional lives separate. You do not want to damage your professional relationship with him, but you do not want to date him. You could escalate your assertion by saying:

EMPATHIC COMPONENT   "I am flattered by your persistence.

DESCRIPTION OF SITUATION   But I have thought about it and have made up my mind.

EXPECTATIONS   I will not change my decision.

POSITIVE CONSEQUENCE   If we could put aside the dating issue, we could enjoy our working relationship."

All further communication about the topic probably would stop. In some instances, "closing the door" on an issue may very well be your goal. This example illustrates that the consequences of escalating in such a manner are serious enough to require careful consideration prior to using this strategy.

The Responsibility Associated with Saying No

Assertive behavior carries with it responsibility and, if possible, fairness. For example, if you have been participating in an unsafe staffing situation for several weeks or months and recently have decided to set limits assertively on your working conditions, it is only fair for you to alert your supervisor of your intentions in advance. A forewarning—including stated expectations, some possible alternatives, and the action you plan to take—means behaving in a responsible and assertive manner. When you anticipate that the short-staffing situation is about to arise again, you may want to approach your supervisor, reiterate your concerns, but this time share what course of action you plan to take if you are the only professional on duty. Conveying a firm and tactful message is important, and following through with your actions is imperative; but you must be sure that you are willing to carry through with your plan before stating it.
You might say to your supervisor:

EMPATHIC COMPONENT   "I realize there are many times when call-offs create short-staffing situations.

DESCRIPTION OF SITUATION	In the past, I have agreed knowingly to work in severely understaffed situations. I have decided that I will no longer contribute to this unsafe patient care by working alone when three nurses are assigned to staff the unit.
EXPECTATIONS	I expect to work with at least one other nurse, preferably two nurses, as scheduled.
POSITIVE CONSEQUENCE	I'll feel a lot better about my work if my assignment is reasonable."
or	
NEGATIVE CONSEQUENCE	"If I see that the staffing continues to be unsafe, I will resign my position."

After informing your supervisor of your assertive stance, it may be advisable to explore the alternatives available. Other creative options to this example of an unsafe staffing situation might be that a P.R.N. pool of float nurses could be organized, or admissions could be reduced. Probably, you will feel better carrying out your plan if you are assured that administration was informed ahead of time and that options were reviewed.

Careful thought to the consequences of your assertive behavior cannot be overemphasized. While it is important to ask yourself "What's the worst that can happen," it would be irrational to focus exclusively on the negative outcome that if you refuse to work without safe staffing quotas, you will lose your job. Be realistic. Plan for how you might cope with that possibility, but do not dwell on that thought. Do not let negative outcomes control you. Once you have planned for the worst, the other possible options will come into view more clearly.

Once you feel more comfortable refusing requests, you will be surprised by how much more understanding you will be when others do the same. A natural reciprocity follows that if you have the right to refuse a request, so does another person. Undoubtedly, you will find yourself feeling freer to make requests of others, knowing that they will say no if they want to do so.

This freedom to make and refuse requests will be reflected in how you approach people and situations. Assertive nurses are positive, self-confident, goal-directed, and in control of their lives. People naturally respond positively to such affirming attitudes, and enriched relationships can result.

Unfortunately, nurses who are not acquainted with the concepts of assertiveness may feel irrationally that assertive people are not warm and sensitive. On the contrary, personal and professional relationships with assertive nurses can be comfortable, authentic, and enriching.

5. IRRATIONAL BELIEF	Assertive individuals are cold and castrating. Others won't like me if I'm assertive.
RATIONAL COUNTER-PART	Assertive individuals are direct and honest, and behave appropriately. They show real concern for others' rights and feelings as well as their own. Assertiveness enriches relationships.

Of course, as you begin to function in a more assertive manner, the character of some of your relationships may change. In some cases, relationships which formerly thrived on dependency and game playing may not respond well to openness and honesty. When this occurs, you can maintain control of your life by choosing the types and degrees of relationships in which to invest; it is certainly not appropriate for all relationships to be of the same intensity. However, because assertive behavior is honest, often the other person in the relationship comes to rely on truthful interchanges and is relieved to find such openness. Such prevailing honesty means that energy is not expended in game playing or avoiding the truth but rather is channeled positively into constructive interaction.

A nursing instructor in a long-term psychiatric setting described the open, honest relationship she had with a physician colleague. On one occasion, she invited him to speak to the students in her class. During his presentation, he explained that some of the patients were receiving experimental drugs. The assertive nurse asked him if patients had given their informed consent to take these medications, and he responded that they had not. After class, the nurse and the physician discussed the matter. The physician asked the nurse's opinion on whether she thought he should have the patients sign a consent form. She advised him first to inform the patients about the risks involved in the drug regime and then to provide them with an opportunity either to refuse or to sign the consent forms. Because the nurse confronted the physician in an assertive manner without attacking him, he was receptive to her suggestions, and they continued to enjoy a working relationship of mutual trust and respect.

Relationships do not always run smoothly, of course. There are times when some uncomfortable feelings are brought forth. One of the most common of these feelings is anger, around which some irrational beliefs are centered.

6. IRRATIONAL BELIEF	If I assert myself, others will get mad at me.
RATIONAL COUNTERPART	They may or may not get mad/ may feel closer to me/may like what I say/may help me to solve the problem.

Often we find ourselves participating in situations or activities that we do not enjoy, out of fear that if we refuse to continue, others will become angry with us. The reality is that they may or may not get angry. They may appreciate an expression of real feelings about the matter and may even end up supporting an alternative suggestion, should we have the courage to make one.

As an example of a family-related situation, assume that Christmas gift giving has been a tradition in your extended family for a number of years. You feel that with the number of relatives increasing continuously, you want to discontinue the gift exchanges except for select relatives. You have made this decision and are satisfied with it; however, you are reluctant to suggest the change out of fear that your relatives will be angry with you. Although it is possible they may get angry, they also may support your idea and welcome a change from the traditional routine. Recognizing the realistic possibility of the latter occurrence, you can proceed with formalizing an approach to your relatives by using the components of the assertive response/approach:

EMPATHIC COMPONENT	"I know we have been exchanging Christmas gifts with each other for years. I've really enjoyed receiving them.
DESCRIPTION OF SITUATION	However, with our increasing numbers, I am finding it more difficult to buy so many presents.
EXPECTATIONS	I would like to continue giving our individual presents to Mom and Dad and to draw names among the rest of us.
POSITIVE CONSEQUENCE	That way, the Christmas preparations will be more enjoyable and less cumbersome for all of us."

Consider now this example of a professional situation: You are a staff nurse working on a medical-surgical unit. You would like to help patients have more social interaction, so you come up with the idea of initiating daily, small-group activities for patients. You are fearful, however, that the other staff members—especially your head nurse—will think your idea is ridiculous. They probably will get angry (irrational belief), you think to yourself, and say, "This is a hospital for sick people, not a recreation center!" While it is true that they might get angry, especially if they feel the organization of such activities would make more work for them, the reality is that they also might like your suggestion and even help you in implementing it (rational counterpart). You will never know how an idea will be received unless you present it.

After planning how you would deal with the possible consequences of your assertion, you may decide to approach your head nurse in this way:

EMPATHIC COMPONENT	"I know that you like us to make suggestions for the improvement of patient care.
DESCRIPTION OF SITUATION	I have been thinking about how beneficial it would be for patients to interact more with each other.
EXPECTATIONS	I would like to organize a daily group activity on the unit. I am willing to suggest the idea at our staff meeting this week and to volunteer to chair a committee to develop it.
POSITIVE CONSEQUENCES	If we could implement this program and include patients in our planning, it would help us to work together for the improvement of patient care."

A second irrational belief related to anger is that if the other person does get angry, it will be intolerable.

7. IRRATIONAL BELIEF	If other people get angry, I will be devastated.
RATIONAL COUNTERPART	I can handle anger without falling apart. Another's anger is not my responsibility. It is his choice to get angry.

When anger is expressed, you do not have to fall apart. The other person certainly has a right to get angry. If he chooses to react in an angry manner, it is his responsibility and his choice.

As a personal example, assume that you recently became divorced and have a 5-year-old son. Your mother-in-law has informed you that it is very important to her to maintain contact with her grandson. She calls you on the phone and requests that your son spend the weekend in her home. You do not want the child to go at this particular time because of the recent upheaval but fear that if you deny her request, she will become angry. You send the child regretfully and later wish you had been assertive. If only you had known what to say!

While it is true that your mother-in-law may have become angry, it is also possible that she would have understood your rationale and accepted your denial of her request. However, whether she would have become angry with you does not have to be of any real consequence in making your decision. You have the right to decide for yourself and your child where the most appropriate place is for him to spend the weekend. Furthermore, if your mother-in-law would have become angry, she certainly had that right. Her reactions and behavior truly would be her choice—over which you do not, and should not, have any control.

If the opportunity occurs another time and you feel similarly, you are now prepared to say something like:

EMPATHIC COMPONENT	"I know how much you want Johnny for the weekend, and I want you to have contact with each other, too.
DESCRIPTION OF SITUATION	But considering all the disruption that has occurred around here lately,
EXPECTATIONS	I want Johnny to stay home this weekend.
POSITIVE CONSEQUENCES	We both need some time to relax and enjoy each other.
OPTIONAL ALTERNATIVE	Perhaps the two of you can get together for awhile next weekend. I will see how things are going then. If you would like, we can talk closer to the time."

Furthermore, you may want to consider establishing some ground rules for the future. Do you want to schedule your child for entire weekends at Grandma's on a routine basis? This may be what Grandma would like, but what about you and your child? Perhaps the visits would be more appropriately left flexible and dependent upon the circumstances and feelings of all concerned.

The second part of the rational counterpart most recently mentioned emphasizes that anger comes from within individuals. Identical situations can provoke anger in one person but not in another. This is concretely illustrated in the following example. A 3-year-old is playing outside. Mother calls him in for lunch. Johnny immediately screams and hollers, throws his toys, and announces that he is not coming in. Did the mother "cause" this angry outburst? Certainly, her call to lunch precipitated it, but the response came from within the child because of the kind of person he is and perhaps also because of the relationship existing between that particular child and his mother. The point is, however, that it was the child's choice to get angry. The mother did not make him respond as he did. He also could have chosen to say, "O.K., Mom. I'm coming," then pick up his toys, and run into the house.

Understanding and accepting this principle can be a big help in providing you with the impetus to be assertive. Once you recognize the significance of the power and control you have over your own feelings and behavior, the easier it will be to act assertively. Likewise, the more you realize the responsibility others have for controlling their actions, the freer you will feel to be assertive with them. No longer will you feel responsible for their behavior. The way another person responds is truly his choice. If he does choose, then, to react angrily to an assertion, you need not be devastated because you can realize that just as you have the freedom to respond in your own way to a given situation, so does he.

Dealing with Another Person's Anger Assertively

You must decide for yourself, of course, how much of another person's anger you are willing or able to tolerate. When you are the recipient of another person's anger, you have the right to evaluate whether, in your opinion, the anger and the manner of its expression are justified. You can certainly express your opinion in an assertive manner and clarify the issue according to your perception. You can also walk away.

For example, a head nurse in a large metropolitan hospital found herself the continual victim of a particular physician's aggressive outbursts. On one occasion, he screamed that an ordered stool specimen had not been done. The nurse recognized the importance of the order and tried to explain the realistic reason for the delay. However, the physician continued his verbal attack in an uncontrollable manner. Eventually, the nurse asserted, "I'm not able to communicate with you when you behave like that. When you calm down and if you would like to discuss the matter further, I'll be in my office." Then she left the area. In this instance, the nurse felt the discussion was futile, and she chose not to tolerate verbal abuse any longer.

In instances where you feel your mistakes or omissions provoke anger in others, you can admit assertively that you are at fault and learn to accept the other person's anger in an assertive way. For example, suppose that you are a head nurse who promised your staff a short time ago that all of them would have two weekends off per month. You are not able to follow through with that promise, and the staff is angry with you. You recognize that they have a right to be angry, but, by the same token, you also have a right to make an error in judgment and to be responsible for the consequences of that error. You can choose to handle the situation assertively by saying to the staff:

EMPATHIC COMPONENT	"I don't blame you for being angry about the scheduling.
DESCRIPTION OF SITUATION AND FEELINGS	I know that I promised all of you two weekends off a month, but that is just not possible. I realize now that it was improper planning on my part, and I feel badly about my error.
EXPECTATIONS	However, I am readjusting the schedule
POSITIVE CONSEQUENCES	so that you can count on every

third weekend off from now on."

Sometimes you may be in a position to make decisions or to communicate the decisions of others, which will not be received well. It is important to realize that because of the nature of the task, you cannot please everybody all the time. People will get angry.

Assume now that as a nursing school dean, you have been informed by your superior that one of your programs is too costly and that certain positions must be cut. Because you are not pleased with that solution, you have been working on other approaches, but at the moment there is no other alternative. You have been as tactful and supportive of your faculty as possible in conveying the necessity for the reduced number of positions. However, some of them are quite angry. What can you do about it? Accept their anger assertively. You might say something like, "I know you're angry, and I can understand why. I feel badly about cutting the positions. I wish I didn't have to terminate anyone, but it must be done."

Notice the use of "I" statements in this approach and the avoidance of the "poor me," or guilt-ridden, approach; rather, this tactic is an understanding, accepting, realistic, and assertive statement. No attempts are made to try to "talk people out of" their angry feelings. There is no need to do that. Recognize that anger is a normal, healthy emotion with varying degrees of intensity. It is O.K. for people to be angry. For many people, once "permission" is granted to express anger, it becomes easier to deal with.

How Does Anger Block Assertiveness?

Anger is frequently one of the major blocks inhibiting assertive functioning. For many individuals, anger is a terrorizing feeling that can result in either the extreme of silent immobilization or aggressive "acting out." A person who becomes immobilized as a result of angry feelings actually may be overreacting to a fear of losing control. This fear of loss of control may be experienced by either the originator of the angry feelings or the recipient.

Like pain, suffering, fear, or sadness, anger is an uncomfortable, unpleasant feeling that many people seek to avoid. Not only do we seek to avoid it because of feelings that it arouses, but we "run" from such feelings because of the messages society has conveyed about the expression of anger. Socialization has taught us that it is not proper or polite to become angry. Anger is thought to be a sign of crudeness and immaturity. In some religions, it is even considered sinful. Once children become adults, "anger is expected to be dealt with more subtly. It is to be controlled, not expressed openly. In fact, adults are not supposed to get angry at all" (Madow, 1972, p. 41). However, if it must be expressed, it is much more acceptable for a man to get angry than a woman. It is not considered "ladylike" for women to express anger. A woman's role, society says, should be that of peacemaker or stabilizer. She should keep things running smoothly without dissension or friction.

Similarly, a traditional role of nurses in health care settings has been one of mediator between the patient, his family, and all the other health care workers. Nurses have had the frequently overwhelming task of "keeping the house in order" and everything in harmony. This situation, combined with the frustration experienced in being treated as a member of a low-status, minority group, has been a tremendous source of anger.

As women, nurses are members of a minority group and, as such, can be considered victims. Victims, a group with low levels of status and power, engage in horizontal violence—that is, they behave aggressively with each other rather than with the higher-status group (Dean, 1978). Many of the conflict situations of nurses involving anger are shared in assertiveness workshops. Often they occur between members of the nursing profession. Could this problem be the result of displaced anger? If anger originates, at least in part, from relationships with higher-status groups, it follows, then, that the anger also must be dealt with on that level.

Recognizing Displaced Anger

For a variety of reasons, people misdirect their anger to a source other than the original precipitator. This tendency to handle a situation by looking for another possible source on whom to blame the anger is called "displacement." It is usually done unconsciously. You may be extremely angry with your superior at work for not supporting your innovative ideas but say that you are angry with your subordinates for not producing according to your expectations. Perhaps it would be beneficial to ask more frequently, "Who am I really angry with and why?" A detailed example of displacement is illustrated in the following situation involving a nursing colleague.

You are angry with a colleague for refusing to exchange time with you so that you could attend an all-day workshop. Consequently, you are "conveniently" unable to attend a particular meeting at which she was counting on you for participation and support. In this situation, it is not necessary or even desirable to confront your colleague directly about your anger. She certainly has a right to refuse to change time with you and to offer no reasons or excuses for her decision. However, it is important to recognize and accept the source of your anger so that, by owning it, you will be able to control it more readily.

Via introspection, you realize that the anger displaced onto your colleague is unrealistic. You discover that you are actually angry at yourself for not planning far enough in advance to permit the exploration of other alternatives, thereby ensuring your time off for the workshop. Madow (1972) says that "a common reason for displacing anger is to avoid humiliating or belittling yourself" (pp. 288–289). Had you recognized this real source of your anger earlier, it may have been easier to control it and avoid the retaliation of not attending your colleague's meeting. Once you recognize the real source of your anger, it is easier to decide how to handle it.

Handling Your Anger Assertively

It is important to recognize the positive aspects of anger. Anger can be a source of energy and, as such, can be channeled effectively to produce accomplishments. It can be the power behind the drives to study, to work, to make ourselves attractive, or to be successful. Even though it may not be appropriate in all situations to express anger directly, it should not be denied to oneself. It is the denial of such feelings to oneself that can create disturbing symptoms (Madow, 1972). In reality, being open, honest, and direct (that is, assertive) with oneself is a necessary prerequisite to being assertive with others.

In addition to recognizing that you are angry, it is necessary to identify both the "real" source as well as the "true" reason for your anger and to determine whether that reason is realistic. In other words, identify the person with whom you are angry and why. By accomplishing this goal, you will be able to control your anger more effectively, thereby handling it more assertively.

Eventually, dealing with your anger is the final step that naturally follows from successful accomplishment of the three preceding ones (Madow, 1972). To review, they are as follows:

1. Recognize and accept the fact that you are angry versus denying it.
2. Identify the "real" source of your anger versus displacing it onto someone or something else.
3. Understand why you are angry and whether your reason is realistic.
4. Deal with your anger realistically.

An initial, necessary consideration in dealing with anger that originates in you is to decide on your goal. You may want to ask yourself these questions:

1. What do I want to accomplish in the situation?
2. Am I interested in maintaining an ongoing relationship with this person, or don't I particularly care about the future relationship?
3. Do I, in fact, want to communicate my anger openly to the person provoking it? (It may not always be appropriate or in your best interest.)
4. If I choose to communicate my anger directly, what might the consequences be? Am I prepared to deal with them?
5. Am I willing to take whatever risk may be involved?

If you are not concerned about your future relationship with the other person, you may choose to unload your anger without regard for its effects. In some situations, your goal may not be to be assertive but rather to be aggressive. Remember, it is your choice!

For example, if you witness a person breaking into your car, your concern is to stop the destructiveness immediately and to prevent further damage to your possessions. You lash out in either a verbal or physical attack. In an entirely different situation, you may wish to maintain channels of communication and an ongoing relationship with the person provoking your anger. In such a case, it is more important to resolve your anger constructively. This objective can be accomplished either by an "indirect" or a "direct" approach. Although a "direct" expression of anger has merit (this is discussed later), it is not always the best solution. Your choice regarding whether to express your anger directly or indirectly should be made after a thorough analysis of the individual situation, with consideration given to the five questions listed earlier.

Indirect Expressions of Anger

If, according to your assessment, it is not satisfactory or practical to express your anger directly, then it may be appropriate to find other alternative, indirect, yet assertive ways of dealing with it, as long as the anger is not denied to yourself. Some possible alternatives are the following:

1. *Channeling the energy that the anger produces in other ways.*

Examples: Physical activities such as sports; intellectual or social pursuits.

2. *Changing the situation that is creating the anger, even if this entails giving up some advantages.*

Example: A course participant who was a registered nurse employed in an occupational health setting found herself constantly undermined by her nursing superior. She felt that her innovative ideas and creativity were being stifled. It seemed that no matter what Mary did, her boss was dissatisfied. Mary appeared to be a very capable nurse, who was probably a threat to her boss. Mary tried a number of approaches with her superior, including direct sharing of her concerns with the hope of altering their relationship. However, when results did not occur, Mary's frustration and anger increased.

She had been motivated to complete college courses for a long time. Consequently, she had numerous university credits, but they had not been directed toward any specific degree. Through implementing the principles of assertiveness, she mobilized her energy (stemming from her anger with her work situation) and made some definite decisions about her professional future. She resigned from her job, entered a collegiate nursing program, and eventually became a satisfied and happy community health nurse.

3. *Making adjustments or adaptations within the situation so that you are able to cope with it better.*

Example: Following an address given by a national legislator at a nursing organization meeting, it was announced that the meeting was open to questions from the audience. A guest of honor, who was the president of a local medical society, immediately took control of the microphone. For an exorbitant amount of time, he gave a rambling rebuttal to the legislator. A particular nurse became increasingly angry at the uncontrollable monopoly of the nursing meeting by the only physician in the room. By recognizing her anger, she was able to control it and use the resultant energy to produce positive results. When others in the group began to stir with irritation and impatience, she attempted to motivate those responsible for the program to set limits on the speaker. When they did not respond and the group became increasingly restless, she stood up and reminded the speaker assertively that according to the agenda, which had been announced, the group was to have an opportunity for direct communication with the legislator. He concluded his remarks, and the program progressed as planned.

Depending on the method of implementation, the selection of any one of the three alternatives just listed can be a potentially assertive yet indirect way of handling anger. Admitting anger is, in itself, being open and honest. Furthermore, taking an active role by using the energy the anger provides to accomplish something positive, instead of passively being a victim of the circumstances by denying or repressing anger, is being assertive.

Direct Expressions of Anger

In certain instances, you may elect to take a more direct approach in expressing anger. As such, your anger will be communicated directly to the person provoking it. This can be accomplished assertively by the following means:

1. *Letting the other person know your feelings without humiliating him.*

This can be done by speaking in "I" statements and directing your anger to the issue or the behavior of the person, whichever is more appropriate, rather than speaking in "you" statements and attacking the individual's personality.

Example: A wife says to her husband regarding his being late for dinner, "I'm really angry about being left with a prepared dinner and not knowing when you were coming home." Compare this response with the following: "You are the most inconsiderate man in the world! Don't you care about anyone else but yourself?"

2. *Letting the other person know clearly and concisely what you expect for the future.*

Example: "When you're going to be more than a half hour late for dinner, I'd appreciate a phone call." Compare this response with the following approach: not stating what you want and having a "cold war" the rest of the evening or setting yourself up for the same situation to repeat itself in the future.

These guidelines can be integrated and used in additional anger-provoking situations such as the following: Suppose you have asked your head nurse repeatedly for your yearly performance evaluation. Although she has been promising it for weeks, it is now a month overdue. Your salary increment is dependent upon it, and you have become increasingly angry over the delay. A possible assertive approach is this one:

EMPATHIC COMPONENT

"I know you've been very busy and have a lot of things on your mind.

DESCRIPTION OF SITUA-
TION AND FEELINGS

But I've asked you a number of times for my performance evaluation. It's now a month overdue. I'm angry about the delay because I really want my salary increment.

EXPECTATIONS

I would like to meet with you for my evaluation conference early next week. Is Monday or Tuesday better for you? [It is wise to build in some opportunity for input by the recipient, if possible, so that she has some choice in the matter as well as some control.]

POSITIVE CONSEQUENCES

I'll feel a lot better receiving the evaluation, not only because of the salary increment but also because it will be helpful for me to know your assessment of my performance."

or

NEGATIVE CONSEQUENCES

"If we do not have the conference by next Tuesday, I will let the supervisor know how I feel."

Because in this particular situation, the staff nurse had not acquired the desired results from previous attempts, it is appropriate to state what action she intends to take (in terms of a negative consequence) if her expectations as stated this time are not met. Whether to state positive or negative consequences, or both, depends upon the specifics involved in a given situation, with each situation requiring evaluation in its own right.

As an example, suppose that you are the nurse in charge of an ambulatory care clinic. On a given morning, appointments are behind schedule, and some patients have been waiting in relatively uncomfortable surroundings on hard benches for well over an hour. A hospital social worker enters the clinic as she often does on Tuesday mornings and, in an arrogant manner, announces to you that she wants to see the doctor. You inform her of the circumstances and suggest that she speak with the physician when the clinic is over at noon. Assuming that she left, you continue with your work. In a short while, you check on the physician to try to speed up progress, and you find him with the social worker, discussing an issue at length. You are quite angry and make up your mind that if they do not finish the conversation in 5 minutes, you will interrupt. They do finish, however, so you approach the social worker as she is leaving the clinic, while the doctor sees another patient. To the social worker, you say:

EMPATHIC COMPONENT	"I know that you wanted to talk with Dr. Jones.
DESCRIPTION OF SITUA-ATION AND FEELINGS	But I'm really angry that you didn't listen when I explained the circumstances of this clinic earlier. These patients have been waiting for over an hour, and some of them two hours, to see the doctor.
EXPECTATIONS	I would appreciate it if you would not interrupt the clinic anymore on Tuesday mornings unless it's an absolute necessity.
POSITIVE CONSEQUENCES	If we could proceed uninterrupted, the patients would be

seen sooner. Also, if you approach Dr. Jones at another
time, he may be in a better position to give you more of his attention."

In addition to dealing with the presenting problem of the interruption by the social worker, it would also be appropriate in the
given situation to do something assertively about the underlying
problem—that is, the hectic pace of the clinic and the length of
time patients are forced to wait. The nurse could suggest an alternative approach to the person responsible for scheduling the patients; or, if the problem centers around the expediency of the
physician, she could also discuss that matter with him assertively
by stating her suggestions for improvement.

It is important to realize that anger can be handled directly in
a constructive way and used for the mutual benefit of everyone involved. Its honest expression can contribute to the authenticity of
a relationship and may free the other person to reciprocate by sharing his real feelings. Direct expressions of anger can be controlled
and need not leave either the recipient or the originator destroyed
or devastated. Furthermore, anger can be expressed directly in an
assertive way. You can express your anger without being mali-
cious and without destroying the other person in the process. You
can be angry and still be assertive.

Buying Time

While it is beneficial to deal with an anger-producing situation, it
is also advantageous to recognize the intensity of your feelings
and give yourself an opportunity to "buy some time" to regain
self-control if you need it to plan a more satisfactory approach. To
do this, you might say, "I'm so furious that I can't even talk about
this now! Let's 'sleep on it' and get together tomorrow morning.
What about 10 A.M. in the Conference Room?" It is wise to be specific about a time and place for a future meeting; otherwise, a
vague "we'll discuss it another time" may never occur. This can be

a very sensible approach, especially if emotions are high and the chances of accomplishing anything constructive are slim.

Of course, some individuals respond to an anger-producing situation without giving it much thought by lashing back immediately with a counterattack. Then there are those who do nothing except to wait and let the episode repeat itself until they simply cannot tolerate it any longer. In frustration, they finally resort to an aggressive attack and often are displeased with themselves and the results.

While self-control and assertiveness are certainly beneficial and worth striving for in anger-producing situations, they are not always possible since, of course, humans are imperfect. However, if you find yourself in a situation in which you have performed in a less desirable way than you would have preferred, evaluate in retrospect the whole process. Learn from it so that you will be equipped to deal with the next situation more effectively.

Unfinished Business

To increase your chances of effectiveness and efficiency, handle an anger-producing situation within a "reasonable" period of time—ideally, from soon after it occurs to within a few days. Otherwise, your energy will be tied up unnecessarily in an unproductive way. If you have found yourself harboring angry feelings for weeks, months, or even years, you know how increasingly difficult it becomes to resolve an issue the longer it has remained in the realm of "unfinished business."

However, waiting does not mean that resolution is impossible. It is not too late to reopen a situation about which you have a lot of anger if, by so doing, you predict that it will make you feel better or increase your chances of resolving the issue. Before you decide to reopen a long-standing issue, you may want to ask yourself some questions:

1. How important is this issue to me?
2. What do I hope to accomplish by getting the issue out in the open?

3. Do the possible benefits of reopening the issue outweigh maintaining the "status quo"? Which will I be content to live with?

4. How can I present my concerns assertively to increase my chances of attaining my goal?

5. What might the possible consequences be? Am I prepared to handle them?

Many of these questions are similar to the ones you may want to reflect on and ask yourself in preparation for being assertive in any situation.

Giving Criticism Assertively

Just as "timing" is an important consideration in dealing with anger, it is also of special significance in handling criticism. When you are in a position to give criticism to another person, give it as soon as possible (within reason) after the incident occurs rather than waiting for hours, days, or months to pass by. Hopefully, the effect of the criticism will be more meaningful that way.

We have all heard mothers reprimanding their children, "Johnny, you shouldn't have done that! Wait until your father comes home!" What kind of message is this giving to the child? On the one hand, it is saying that Daddy has more clout and is perhaps better able to handle the situation than Mother, which may or may not be true. It is also saying that the situation (and likewise the child) is not important enough to deal with now and can be delayed until later. If the incident is significant enough to warrant criticism, then it is also important enough to handle more promptly. Often anger and criticism go hand-in-hand. When you are in a situation evoking criticism, you may also be angry with the person involved. Some guidelines to use when giving criticism are as follows:

1. Be direct and specific. Speak in "I" statements.

2. Do not criticize the person; rather, identify the behavior with which you are dissatisfied.

3. State the criticism in a positive manner by explaining your expectations.

As an example, a charge nurse might tell her staff, "I was not pleased with the condition of the office yesterday at the end of the shift. The charts were scattered all over the place. Before you go off duty today, I want the office put in order and the charts placed in their racks." Compare this type of criticism with the following aggressive one: "You people have a lot of nerve leaving this office the way you did yesterday. Haven't you ever learned to put things away when you're finished with them? You'd better not leave this place a mess again."

By way of another example, suppose you received your performance evaluation a few days ago from your head nurse, and it was very positive overall. While in the nurses' station this morning, a practical nurse co-worker made a comment which revealed that she had seen your written evaluation. You are angry with the head nurse for leaving it exposed and available to other staff because you believe that performance evaluations should be confidential. You decide to be assertive by letting your head nurse know your criticism and what you expect:

EMPATHIC COMPONENT	"Even though your intention may not have been to leave out my performance evaluation for others to see,
DESCRIPTION OF SITUATION AND FEELINGS	I am aware that it has been read by a certain staff member. I am angry about that because I expected it to be kept confidential.
EXPECTATIONS	In the future, I would like it kept in a secure place so other staff members will not have access to it."

Further consider this example: You are the nurse in charge of a long-term psychiatric ward this evening. You are aware that the two attendants assigned to the unit are reluctant to work and often spend a significant portion of their shift either watching television or reading magazines. You have never worked with them before, so you communicate specifically to each of them their tasks for the evening. Within a half hour, you see one of them sitting in the lounge area alone, reading a magazine. You decide to approach him in a kind but firm manner:

EMPATHIC COMPONENT	"Although it might be hard for you to get going this evening, John, there is a lot of work to be done around here and that is what we are getting paid to do.
EXPECTATIONS	I'd like you to distribute clean towels and soap now to each patient on your ward in preparation for baths or showers later on. That will also give you the opportunity to greet the patients, see how they're doing, and decide who needs you to spend time with them before dinner.
POSITIVE CONSEQUENCES	If we all do our share, the work will get done and the patients will receive good care."

In this particular situation, it is important to emphasize firmly, yet tactfully, what you expect John's work performance to be rather than attacking and undermining him as a person by remarks such as these: "I should have known better than to accept being in charge of a shift with you on it. I was warned about your laziness. What do you think you're getting paid for anyhow? Certainly not to read magazines. Now get moving, and get some work done."

Hopefully, the former, assertive approach will not only encourage John to produce but will also help the nurse to gain his respect. Another important factor here is that the nurse conveyed her criticism and expectations the first time she was exposed to John's unpredictable behavior. She did not let incident after incident occur before setting limits, which could have increased her chances of becoming aggressive.

Receiving Criticism Assertively

When you are on the receiving end of another's criticism, you may want to consider the following:

1. *Evaluate the source.*

Do you have much respect for the person giving the criticism? Do you value his opinion? Have you heard the same criticism before? If so, the chances of it being accurate are greater, and perhaps it would be in your best interest to take it seriously.

2. *Ask for clarification.*

If you are criticized for your lack of "leadership ability," you have a right to ask for more specifics, with examples, of what is meant.

3. *If you feel the criticism is unfair, say so.*

You have a right to give your opinion. On a written performance evaluation, you may also want to include your comments in writing.

4. *If you feel the criticism is justified, you can accept it assertively.*

You do not have to apologize for human errors like making a mistake or forgetting to do something. For instance, suppose a particular employee requested a day off. You agreed to accommodate her but forgot to include the request in the completed schedule. When you are criticized for your omission, you can handle the situation by sticking to the issue and ignoring whatever personal comments may be made about your ability. Saying something like the following would be appropriate: "You're right, Julie. I did say you could have next Thursday off. I'll make the necessary adjustment on the schedule right now. I'm glad you called it to my attention."

Handling Put-downs Assertively

Criticism in its most negative form can be referred to as a "put-down." The intent of a put-down is to humiliate or to demean the other person in an attempt to boost the image of its initiator. The overall goal in responding to a put-down is to counter its intent by saying something in an open, honest way that makes you feel good about yourself. By so doing, conclude the discussion of the issue rather than retorting with sarcasm or perpetuating the caustic remarks. Consider this example:

PUT-DOWN: "I don't know how your staff stands you!"

RESPONSE: "They think I'm terrific!"

If the put-down catches you by surprise and you are at a loss for words, you might want to respond with a comment that will take the attention off yourself and focus it on the other person temporarily, thus giving you time to think of an appropriate remark. A way to do this is by saying, "You must have had a reason for saying that..." or "Tell me what you mean by that..." Also, you can ask for the remark to be repeated, saying something like "What was that?" or "Run that by me again..." This can help to call attention to the inappropriateness of the remark so that the speaker may not repeat it. In that way, the put-down can be terminated as a topic of conversation.

If you can identify put-downs that you receive repeatedly, you may want to take some time to think of a "pat" response that makes you feel good about yourself, which you will be prepared to use as needed. Some examples are given here:

PUT-DOWN:	"What's a pretty girl like you doing unmarried?"
RESPONSE:	"It's marvelous to have so much freedom."

. . . .

PUT-DOWN:	"And when do you plan to start your family?"
RESPONSE:	"We're thoroughly enjoying our twosome."

. . . .

PUT-DOWN:	(Said sarcastically) "It must be nice to make all that money!"
RESPONSE:	"It does have its advantages."

. . . .

PUT-DOWN:	Your height has been a target of jokes. Frequently, you hear "How's the air up there?"
RESPONSE:	"Terrific—it's pollution-free."

. . . .

PUT-DOWN:	Being short, you're frequently called "Shorty" and offered a chair to stand on or someone else's assistance, which you do not want.
RESPONSE:	"Thanks for the offer, but I prefer getting it myself."

Some specific put-downs that nurses receive are illustrated here along with some possible responses:

PUT-DOWN	(Said sarcastically by a physi-

| | cian) "I thought part of your job was to follow orders. Oh, that's right—nurses *think* these days." |
| RESPONSE: | "Yes, we're really very capable." |

. . . .

| PUT-DOWN: | Upon introduction, a co-worker says, "Oh, you're one of those B.S.N. grads!" |
| RESPONSE: | "I plan to use my education to help us all work well together." |

. . . .

| PUT-DOWN: | (From a physician) "I'm glad to hear you're trying to educate nurses. Anything you could do would be an improvement." |
| RESPONSE: | "The profession is making great strides." |

. . . .

| PUT-DOWN: | (From a patient to an L.P.N. nursing student) "Last night I had a private-duty nurse, and now I have to settle for a 'student' and a 'practical' nurse student at that!" |
| RESPONSE: | "Sounds like you received good care last night. I plan to give you good care today, too." |

Other times you will find it best just to bypass the put-down and stick to the issue at hand. For instance, when confronted by a co-worker who makes the remark, "Oh, I can see it must be your time of the month," you may want to respond by saying, "My hormonal system has nothing to do with the issue at hand." Then proceed to state what you want. For example, "I prefer to have our discussion focus on Mrs. Smith's care."

Although the natural response to a put-down is to retort with either aggression or sarcasm, you can be effective and feel much better about yourself if you can control these behaviors. Remember that the objective in responding to a put-down is not to continue the discussion of that topic but rather to say something that enhances your self-esteem. The more positive you feel about yourself, the easier it is to be assertive.

How Does Anxiety Relate to Assertiveness?

Just as self-confidence and repeated successful encounters contribute to increased assertions, the presence of "blocks" such as those previously mentioned (irrational beliefs, anger, criticism, and put-downs) tends to inhibit one's ability to function assertively. An additional "block" which must be addressed is anxiety.

Suppose it is 3:00 A.M. and you are working the 11:00 P.M.-to-7:00 A.M. shift at a college student health service. A student has come in with symptoms that you feel should be checked by a physician that night. Although there is a physician "on call," he has made it quite clear that he does not expect to be awakened during the night. He lives nearby but feels that all "emergencies" should be taken to the local hospital emergency room or wait until morning. You disagree with his directive. In spite of the fact that the college assures parents of on-campus medical attention 24 hours a day, this student would have to find transportation and possibly pay emergency room fees.

As you walk to the telephone to place the call, you remember the last time you had to phone this physician in the middle of the night. That night he berated you for awakening him. Because you were flustered and could not think straight, the facts came out garbled. As his voice got louder and louder, you felt smaller and smaller. Your passive responses intensified his anger. As you now recall that conversation, the uneasiness returns. You can feel the apprehension and queasiness creeping over you. Your stomach churns as you dial the physician's number, pondering what to say.

This is an example of how anxiety impedes assertive behavior. The more you worry about what will happen, the more tense you become. When anxiety blocks your assertive behavior, you are often displeased with how you handle the interaction. This same chain of events can occur repeatedly.

Anxiety can be overcome at the time it occurs by countering it with assertive behavior through the use of the following three approaches (Bloom, Coburn, and Pearlman, 1975).

1. *Imagine a successful assertion.*

You could imagine yourself confidently calling the physician, giving him a report of the patient's condition without conveying an apologetic message. You can think about the various positive outcomes of your successful assertion: "This time when I approach the physician in a forthright manner, he may be more cognizant of his responsibilities. He may be appreciative of the report. He may even be cordial."

2. *Use covert messages or self-encouragement.*

You could give yourself covert messages as you walk to the telephone and dial the physician's number. These messages might include: "I'll feel better about the patient after I have called the physician" or "I have a right to call the physician regarding this student's condition. The reality is that this doctor is on call." Further, "The physician is also responsible for the student's health, and I have a right to notify him" or "The student has a right to the on-campus medical care as promised by the college."

3. *Practice conscious relaxation.*

As you anticipate the assertion, you could practice a conscious relaxation technique such as deep abdominal breathing. This is one of several approaches to relaxing the body systematically to ease tension and anxiety. Other ways to relax the body and mind (such as yoga, transcendental meditation, and progressive relaxation exercises) are covered extensively in other texts. Assertive behavior flows more readily from a relaxed body and mind.

Another way to reduce anxiety or prevent its build-up is through advanced planning, when the situation lends itself to preparation ahead of time. Planning can include gathering more information, reviewing what you are going to say in your own mind, writing it out on paper, or rehearsing it with a friend. Planning is discussed further in Chapter 6, but it is important at this point to recognize its relationship to anxiety reduction.

Anxiety can also be a positive influence by serving as a clue to the need for assertive behavior and providing the impetus for action. Recognizing the physical symptoms that may result from an anxiety-producing situation can help you in this respect. For example, suppose that your boss announces to you in the late afternoon that you are to give an hour presentation the following morning which, by its nature, will take considerable preparation time. You are so taken back by the abrupt and forceful manner in which the assignment was given that you accept it passively. The more you think about it, though, the more angry and anxious you become. In fact, during the preparation time, you develop a throbbing headache and have difficulty sleeping that night. In the morning, you can hardly eat breakfast, and you find yourself experiencing episodes of diarrhea.

Other physical symptoms that can be manifestations of anxiety include blushing, a rapid heart rate, nail biting, constipation, an increased appetite, cramps, and nausea. When you find yourself experiencing any combination of these symptoms, it can be helpful to ask yourself, "What is my body reacting to? Should I have been assertive?" Although these symptoms can result from a number of physical and emotional conditions, their presence can signal a lack of assertiveness and alert you to the need for assertive behavior.

In the situation involving the last-minute assignment, the employee could respond to her boss assertively in a variety of ways:

1. Tactfully but firmly refuse the assignment as given, indicating that she needs more preparation time to do a competent job. Suggest her willingness to give the presentation if the meeting can be changed to a later date.
2. Indicate her willingness to present the material, explain-

ing that due to the short notice, she will need the help of
two other employees to gather and compile the data.

3. Convey the realistic inconvenience presented by the timing of the assignment but indicate willingness to do it if
   some compensation can be received in return (for example,
   more money for overtime preparation or extra time off).

You Can Overcome Blocks to Assertiveness

Coping successfully with anxiety is a crucial step in learning to
function assertively because often important situations in which
we really want to behave assertively are also anxiety producing.
Although assertive behavior can be learned and developed through
practice, it is not always easy to achieve, especially when "blocks"
or "inhibitors" such as the ones described in this chapter are present. However, their existence is typical in that they are a usual
part of the human experience. Remember that they can be overcome through practicing the techniques discussed in this chapter.
Indeed, their mastery serves as a challenge to all nurses seeking
continued refinement of assertive skills!

References

Bloom, Lynn, Karen Coburn, and Joan Pearlman. *The New Assertive
    Woman.* New York: Dell, 1975.
Dean, Patricia Geary. Towards Androgeny. *Image* 10(1) (1978):10–14.
Ellis, Albert, and R. A. Harper. *A Guide to Rational Living.* North Holly-
    wood, Calif.: Wilshire Book Company, 1974.
Madow, Leo. *Anger: How to Recognize and Cope with It.* New York:
    Charles Scribner's Sons, 1972.

6

Promoters of Assertiveness

The preceding chapter discusses the various blocks to assertive behavior and ways to overcome inhibiting forces. Because assertiveness focuses on the positive, a discussion is appropriate regarding those factors and activities that enhance and promote assertive behavior. Promoters of assertive behavior vary from internal feelings of self-confidence to external techniques of writing out scripts and role playing. This chapter emphasizes promoters such as anticipation and planning, as well as various skill-building techniques.

Not all the suggested promoters will be helpful to you, but at least one may be the missing element you need to enhance your assertive techniques and increase the frequency of your successful assertions. While not all situations warrant assertive behavior and while assertiveness does not guarantee success, as you increasingly adopt an assertive philosophy or attitude, you will feel better about yourself and your life. Therefore, the promoters discussed in this chapter can become not only promoters of assertive behavior but also promoters of a more positive and rewarding life-style.

The Cyclic Effect of Successful Assertions

In order for nurses to function assertively as often as they desire, positive assertive behavior must be initiated and reinforced. Once you begin to assert yourself and feel good about your successes, your anxiety about future assertions will lessen. This process naturally reinforces you to be assertive again (Bloom, Coburn, and Pearlman, 1975). Development of self-confidence in assertions is why you should make your first assertive attempts in low-risk situations where you have a greater chance of success and where failure, if it does occur, is not likely to be devastating. You can select the kinds of situations as well as the time and place to be assertive by purposefully structuring experiences that are likely to yield positive results. These successful assertions promote confidence, and confidence, in turn, promotes more successful assertions. In fact, such a positive cycle in itself becomes a promoter of assertive behavior. Likewise, such behavior is reinforced by anticipation and planning.

The Art of Anticipating

Often nurses report that they think of what they could have said assertively after an incident has occurred, or they accept responsibility and then later resent the decision or commitment that was made. They ask, "Will I ever be able to be assertive 'on the spot'?" The answer is yes. With practice, your assertions will become more spontaneous. As you become more aware of opportunities to be assertive, the time period between the incident and your awareness of how to deal with it assertively will become shorter. Soon the assertive awareness "click" will occur during the incident. Eventually, you will reach the point where you anticipate incidents or their outcomes and plan your assertive approach or response accordingly. A simple example of this process follows.

You have taken a screen door to the hardware store for repair, explaining that you must have it back by the following Saturday for a big party. The store clerk assures you that it will be repaired and ready for pick-up Saturday morning. Because you have never had anything repaired at this store before, you do not know if the assurance is reliable. In anticipation of possible problems, you decide that it would be wise to ask the clerk's name and call her a few days in advance to remind her of your deadline. This is one way for you to anticipate possible negative outcomes and prevent a disappointment later.

"But," you may ask, "how can I anticipate or predict what might happen?" In general, you can learn to anticipate outcomes by keeping well informed and, more specifically, by carefully "tuning in" to others. One aspect of anticipating in the professional arena is knowing organizational expectations and legal constraints. There are two main areas of information to consider: (a) your organization's policies and union contract, if applicable; and (b) your state's Nurse Practice Act.

A union contract or organizational policy does not need to constrain your assertions completely, but you should consider the risks involved. For example, if the contract under which you work calls for assigned dinner hours and you see flexible dinner hours as a solution to a staffing problem, you need to weigh the problems you will encounter by proposing flexible dinner hours against other alternative solutions. Practices that are in violation of a union contract are not easy to execute and thus should be worth the effort of an assertion. You may need to find another interim solution until the next contract is negotiated, at which time you can act assertively to encourage change. Regardless of whether you are covered by a contract, it is equally important for you to be cognizant of the policies of the organization for which you work. Violating organizational policies has certain consequences, and you need to be aware of them in order to make assertive decisions about your behavior.

As a nurse, you have the right to practice nursing within the scope of the Nurse Practice Act of the state in which you work. Because Nurse Practice Acts vary from state to state, understanding the act of your state is crucial when asserting professional rights, for it sets the legal limits of your practice. If you want to do something outside the scope of your Nurse Practice Act, then your assertive efforts should focus on changing the act or its rules and regulations.

Another way of keeping informed of professional issues and activities is to create a network of colleagues who share appropriate information informally on a regular basis or specifically upon request. (Networks are discussed further in Chapter 7.) An increased awareness of your environment will help you to anticipate potential outcomes more accurately and to choose appropriate responses.

Some situations, however, cannot be anticipated by keeping generally informed of issues or affairs; rather, they require you to "tune in" to another person. Without negating the principle of an individual's choice of response, paying close attention to the other

person's values and behavior will sharpen the acuity of your pre-
dictions and enable you to plan accordingly. For example, if you
want to approach your boss about a nagging personnel problem,
you will want to be sensitive to his cues. Perhaps he is trying to
meet some deadline or is having a bad day. If, to your knowledge,
you have chosen the most appropriate time and have paid careful
attention to his previous responses in similar situations, you should
have a fairly accurate idea of his position on issues of this nature.
Therefore, you will know the types of opposition you may encounter and can be prepared to present your facts and rationale accordingly.

Anticipating and planning often go hand-in-hand, especially
in high-risk assertions. Ideally, you will want to plan for success by
learning to take advantage of opportunities and to counter objec-
tions with appropriate information, even if it means rescheduling
encounters. For example, if you are supposed to present a report at
a meeting and you learn that some essential information will not
be available in time to be included in the report, an assertive approach would be either to alter the agenda or to reschedule the
meeting.

On other occasions, you may want to anticipate and plan for
the human element of an encounter. For instance, if your report
identifies the weaknesses of a specific department, you may want
to have the necessary data to support your conclusions as well as a
plan for how you will respond if the recipient of the report becomes
upset or defensive. A preplanned possible response with some
built-in flexibility can increase your chances of handling the situation effectively.

As you master assertive skills and use them more often, you
will start to anticipate incidents and their outcomes naturally.
Sometimes planning will be simultaneous; at other times, you will
need to anticipate so that planning can begin.

Planning: Time Well Spent

Nurses plan patient care, and they help patients plan how to integrate health care into their life-styles. Thus, it is commonly accepted that nurses must plan and be organized in order to complete

the many complex tasks they perform daily. This assumption is especially strong in light of the fact that most nurses are busy people, usually women juggling full- or part-time jobs and family responsibilities. However, there is an important difference between being "organized" in order to get things done and accurately defining what needs to be done and how it might be accomplished most effectively as part of the "planning" process.

Admittedly, nurses do plan and are organized, but these activities are usually "other directed." In other words, nurses make decisions based on what is best for patients, their spouses, their families, or their employers, with little attention to their own rights, needs, and desires. Unfortunately, many nurses do not transfer the principles of planning to themselves. For example, traditionally, nurses have viewed their careers as temporary, secondary to the goals of marriage and a family. In addition to such personal factors, nursing has been considered an action-oriented profession. Nurses are expected to be on the move, to be busy "doing things" rather than thinking and planning. Where does it say on a typical assignment sheet "plan for tomorrow," or next month, or next year? Indeed, most nurses do not plan their lives or their careers, much less their assertions.

Planning your assertions can increase your chances of getting what you want and can help you to feel good about yourself. When you plan an assertion, you identify what you want, what you are going to say, and how you are going to say it. In addition, you consider the possible consequences, including how the other person might respond.

While planning has relevance to day-to-day situations and assertions, it is also used by the assertive nurse to set the direction for her personal and professional life. In this respect, the typical nurse has drifted in and out of the profession or from job to job without much purposeful planning and forethought. While certainly it is the individual nurse's choice to determine the extent to which she wants to be involved in her profession and how seriously she wishes to consider her career, many nurses are not even aware of the value of career planning. Consequently, they end up midway or at the end of their careers wishing that they had done things differently.

To a degree, this situation is reflective of the fact that the majority of nurses are women. Women are less likely than men to develop a career plan, and, subsequently, when they finally establish the priorities of their ambitions, it is virtually impossible to achieve them. Unlike men, women put themselves at a disadvantage by not having firm, clear goals to identify exactly what they want to do, where they want to do it, how much they want to make, and when and how they expect to get there (Foxworth, 1980).

The assertive nurse is different. She realizes that she is the prime mover in her life and is attuned to the advantages of planning her assertions and her life. Career and life planning means figuring out exactly what you want to do and developing and implementing a plan to do it. Such planning, of course, involves being flexbile and open enough to adapt and modify the plan as your needs, goals, or circumstances change. The assertive, career-oriented nurse plans to develop solid competencies first and to become proficient in a given area before searching out new and more challenging tasks. By trying to avoid the subordinate role too quickly, she can miss out on an important step in career development. In addition, the assertive nurse recognizes the value of aiding her subordinates in their career development. By preparing her own replacement, she not only helps the subordinate but also plans for her own progress so that when the opportunity for advancement presents itself, she is free to move upward.

Within the career and life-planning process, you define your whole life mission, your life role, and your lifelong identity (Bolles, 1972). You may find it helpful to ask yourself the following questions:

1. What was my original reason for selecting and entering the nursing profession?
2. Have I accomplished what I originally set out to do a number of months or years ago?
3. Am I in the process of accomplishing my goals?
4. Have I changed my reasons for practicing nursing? If so, why?
5. What do I want to be doing personally and professionally 5 years from now; 10 years from now; at the end of my career?

6. What will it take to get there?

By answering these questions, you place yourself in a better position to acquire and maintain control over your own life. Assertive people do not wait for others to meet their needs or solve their problems. Rather, they enjoy a certain degree of pride in knowing that they are responsible for achieving their own personal and professional goals.

Such was the case with Irene. Like many other nurses, she had chosen a nursing career because, at the time, it provided security and was an acceptable choice for a young woman interested in furthering her education. Her original hopes of working with patients and families in depressed areas soon was diverted by marriage and a family. For 15 years, Irene worked in nursing and raised her family. During this period, she came to enjoy working with patients who had long-term care needs. Recently, however, she had become discontent with her professional life but was unsure of the origin of the problem. Initially she had thought that her problem related to her relationship with her head nurse and the fatigue of working shifts. Further probing uncovered the fact that her discontent ran deeper: Actually, she was troubled by the fact that the unit's constant patient turnover prevented her from developing relationships with patients that she felt were so important to her nursing practice.

In addition, Irene's personal life was changing. With a rapidly maturing family, Irene needed to plan for future educational expenses; further, she was faced with the question of where she would be working in 5 to 10 years. This led Irene to do some introspection and to determine what she really wanted based on her values: Did she want to continue to work with patients in an acute care facility; did she want a higher salary, additional fringe benefits, or a more flexible work schedule? She had to decide how important each of these considerations was to her, not necessarily to others.

While Irene was the most appropriate person to make decisions about her own career, she may have wanted to seek assistance from others, perhaps even pursuing a mentor. A mentor is someone you trust, admire, and respect, who can provide you with career guidance. Although sometimes such relationships evolve naturally, you have the right to seek assistance with your career in an active way by purposefully developing a mentor relationship. The key is your orchestration of the resources.

Another aspect of being a self-determiner is to control the extent to which you permit the past to affect the present. By freeing yourself from aspects of the past that are binding or restrictive, you can live more fully in the present and move into the future. You can do this by responding to the "shoulds" and "shouldn'ts" of the past with "why?" or "why not?" Once the experiences of the past have been put in perspective, the planning process can continue.

Irene came to terms with her past and eventually decided that a nurse practitioner role would help her to move closer to her goal of a more autonomous and accountable role, while still giving her the opportunity to provide direct patient care and to have long-term relationships with patients. Irene then asked herself, "What do I need to do to move from a staff nurse position into a nurse practitioner role?" Gathering credible information is important in the planning process. In Irene's case, she proceeded to interview nurse practitioners, their employers, and nurse educators in order to determine the necessary credentials for obtaining a practitioner position.

Given Irene's extensive experience, she may have already possessed some of the skills required. Depending on the type of position she wanted, additional formal education may or may not have been required. But she would not have been able to make an informed decision unless she determined what skills were required, conducting an honest self-appraisal and assertively seeking to have other people recognize her skills. By identifying her competencies and having confidence in her ability to use them, she was more likely to have others recognize and reward her strengths.

Once Irene evaluated the advantages and disadvantages of either a new job or returning to school and once she determined if the risks were worth taking, she could develop and select an appropriate strategy for accomplishing her goal. Part of the plan might have included convincing a potential employer that she was the right person for the job or the admissions committee of a school that she was an acceptable student. Whatever route Irene selects, her chances of success and self-satisfaction are greatly enhanced by taking the time to plan.

Skill-Building Techniques

Having information, planning, and anticipating all help to promote the actual assertion. The process, however, must culminate in action. Skill-building techniques are discussed here to help you put your plans into action.

Techniques that can help you to function more assertively include role playing, avoiding procrastination, being persistent, building in trial periods, finding and becoming a role model, using the components and writing scripts, and using audiovisual equipment. Although the use of these techniques cannot guarantee assertive behavior, they certainly will support your assertive efforts.

Role Playing

Often the hesitancy to proceed with an assertion is overcome with the practice gained in role playing. Practice will build your confidence, develop your skills, and enhance your effectiveness. Practicing assertive words will decrease your anxiety and help the words to flow naturally in actual situations. Additionally, role playing provides the advantage of allowing you to try several different approaches ahead of time and choosing which one is most desirable and comfortable for you. Having a friend receive your assertion and respond to it can give you the opportunity to practice carrying on an assertive dialogue and to learn how to respond to a variety of retorts.

Avoiding Procrastination

Procrastination can inhibit assertiveness. Sometimes people procrastinate in hopes that the problem will solve itself or that someone else will take action. Often such passive behavior creates exactly what the passive person does not want: more problems.

As an example, Mary Jane, a nurse in one of our assertive training groups, explained that her husband had lost his job 9 months earlier, with the result that she had become their sole support. During the first few months of his unemployment, when he was not looking for a job, she was irritated but "didn't want to say anything." So she remained quiet and told herself that he needed some time to "sort out" his feelings. She kept hoping that he would sense her irritation and begin a job search. By the fourth month she felt overburdened as the only wage earner in the family but still procrastinated in telling him how she felt. By not dealing with her feelings and the situation as they developed, she allowed her tension level to build until, finally, after 6 months with the situation unchanged, Mary Jane experienced an aggressive outburst and threatened to leave her husband if he did not get a job. In class, she reported feeling terrible about how she had handled the whole situation. Through analyzing the situation, she could see that her procrastination had not been helpful.

Some suggestions on what to do about procrastination include recognizing it early and setting deadlines. Reflect on how you have approached or responded to recent situations. Have you put off talking with people about issues or following up on problems? Develop the habit of establishing deadlines for yourself and others. Most people respond positively to a time limit, especially if it is mutually agreed upon. Consider the possible consequences if Mary Jane had said the following to her husband within the first few months of his unemployment:

EMPATHIC COMPONENT	"Herb, I know it was an awful blow when they closed the service department and you lost your job.
DESCRIPTION OF FEEL-INGS AND SITUATION	But I'm feeling discouraged by the uncertainty of this period and being the only wage earner. I think it would be easier for me if I had some idea of how long you think a job search will take.
EXPECTATIONS	I'd like for us to set some deadlines jointly and make contingency plans.

POSITIVE CONSEQUENCES	I'll feel a lot better when we've done that."

Sometimes you may be trying very hard to change nonproductive behavior, but you may find yourself in difficult circumstances and involved with others who also procrastinate. Such situations require perseverence and persistence.

Being Persistent

Nonassertive individuals easily take no for an answer and, at the slightest indication of a negative response, give up and say, "Oh, well . . . I tried." Although this approach avoids conflict and confrontation, it also explains why nonassertive people often fail to get things done. An assertive person is able to distinguish between a firm no and another's indecision, and will respond accordingly. For example, when an assertive nurse gets a firm no to a request, she can still leave the door open for a decision reversal without compromising her own self-esteem.

Let us say that you have requested some new equipment for your department, and the request has been denied. Although you offered several alternatives to assure cost-effectiveness, your boss was not receptive. You can accept that decision assertively and still convey your disappointment, hoping for a decision reversal by saying:

EMPATHIC COMPONENT	"I understand your hestitancy to buy that new expensive equipment.
DESCRIPTION OF FEELINGS	But I want you to know that I'm disappointed.
EXPECTATIONS	I'm willing to help in whatever way I can in order to have the equipment. Let me know if there's anything I can do."

If the recipient of the request does not give a clear yes or no, the assertive nurse will be persistent in finding out what is required to change that indecision to a yes. The assertive nurse might say something like, "I've been asking you about the new equipment for several months, and it seems that you are indecisive. What can I do or what information can I provide to help you make a decision?"

In instances when you do not receive an answer of any kind, you may find the following points helpful to consider:

1. Do not assume automatically that no answer at all equates with a negative response. If possible, wait it out. There may be reasons of which you are not aware that are prohibiting the other person from responding.

2. If you absolutely must have an answer, you may want to give the other person a deadline, as follows:

DESCRIPTION OF SITUATION AND FEELINGS	"I have to let the purchasing department know by the fifteenth of the month if we are going to buy the new equipment. You know that I feel strongly about our need for the new equipment, and in the past you have been supportive of my concerns. But I need your approval to order the equipment.
EXPECTATIONS	We have a meeting scheduled for the thirteenth. I'll need your decision by then."

3. Depending on your relationship with the person, you may want to phrase the deadline in such a way that it becomes the responsibility of the other person to inform you if he does not agree. For example:

DESCRIPTION OF SITUATION	"As you requested, I'm submitting a copy of the final supple-

	mentary budget that is to be sent to Mrs. Winters. I have incorporated my recommendation for the new equipment.
EXPECTATIONS	Unless I hear from you by next Tuesday, I'll assume that you agree, and I'll have the secretary type it."

4. Depending on the nature of the situation, you may want to remind the other person on a regular basis of your request. For example:

EMPATHIC COMPONENT	"I realize I must be sounding like a broken record,
DESCRIPTION OF SITUATION	but every time I prepare a quarterly report, I get enthused about buying that new equipment.
EXPECTATIONS	I'd like to discuss it with you."

5. There comes a time when you have to determine how appropriate it is to continue to be persistent because inappropriate persistence can be destructive. Learn to recognize when an issue is dead. For example, after a reasonable period of not getting the approval, be realistic. Obviously, your boss does not want your department to have the equipment or does not consider it important enough to locate the resources. At this point, you have to decide how important the equipment is to you. If you decide that your department can function without it, you can close the issue in an assertive manner by saying:

DESCRIPTION OF SITUATION	"During the last year, I have asked repeatedly for that new equipment.
EXPECTATIONS	Even though I'd still like it, we have been able to operate without it.

POSITIVE CONSEQUENCES   If you should decide to approve
the expenditure, I'd be pleased."

Building in Trial Periods

As discussed earlier, assertive nurses are willing to take risks. One
way to promote taking a chance is to set limits assertively regarding the consequences of making a mistake. This can be achieved by
building in trial periods when appropriate, as shown in the following example.

Suppose that you have developed a creative way of restruc-
turing and running your department. You are not sure if it will be
more effective than the current status, but you would like to try it.
This is a fairly high-risk situation because failure of the project
could cause multiple problems for staff and patients. For this reason, implementing the new system should include certain built-in
parameters, as follows:

1. Getting staff support and participation in the planning,
   implementation, and evaluation phases.
2. Making it a trial period or demonstration project with
   specific time limits. (It is important that a "demonstration" project or "acting" appointment not continue indefinitely.)
3. Developing evaluation criteria against which the project
   will be measured at a specific time.

Using the Components and Writing Scripts

Another promoter of assertive behavior is to become familiar with
assertive speech. Although each person's communication style is
unique, nurses do well when they have some guidelines for reference in developing their assertive statements.

It is helpful, for instance, to memorize the components of the
assertive response/approach (as outlined by Bloom, Coburn, and

Pearlman, 1975). With these phrases set firmly in their minds, nurses report increased confidence in their ability to use the components to respond assertively or to develop their own assertive style. As introduced in Chapter 1, these components are as follows:

EMPATHIC COMPONENT	"I understand"/"I hear you"
DESCRIPTION OF SITUATION OR FEELINGS	"I feel"/"The situation is"
EXPECTATIONS	"I want"/"The situation requires"
CONSEQUENCES (POSITIVE OR NEGATIVE)	"If you do"/"If you don't"

A natural extension of memorizing the components is to write out the specifics of what you intend to say in a given situation. Many people find that putting the exact words on paper ahead of time helps. For people who are not quite sure what to say in some standard situations, various assertive scripts have been developed and published (Bower and Bower, 1976; Smith, 1975). However, taking the time and energy to write your own scripts by using the "components" as guidelines probably will have more durable and satisfying effects.

Using Audiovisual Aids

As discussed in Chapter 4, assertive words or scripts are not sufficient in themselves. Your voice and body language also must convey assertive messages. Helpful tools to develop these skills include tape recorders, mirrors, and video cameras. Practicing your assertive scripts with a tape recorder can help you to determine if your tone, inflection, and rate are as assertive as the words you select. It is amazing how different a response sounds when it is played back on a tape recorder. Likewise, practicing your assertions in front of a mirror or filming an incident helps you to understand the implications of your body language.

As you rehearse your assertive scripts, evaluate the different parts of your body separately. Are your eyes conveying an assertive message? How about your posture, your arms, your hands?

Using the Assertive Checklist

Finally, a suggested way to integrate many of these promoters with the concepts of assertiveness presented in the earlier chapters of this book is to use the Assertive Checklist (Bloom, Coburn, and Pearlman, 1975). Although the checklist does not lend itself to on-the-spot assertive responses, referring to the questions can be very helpful when planning an assertion in advance. It is an ideal way to assure that you have analyzed the situation from an assertive viewpoint. Ask yourself the following questions when planning an assertion:

1. Have I clarified the situation and focused on the issue? Am I listening to what's being said to validate my understanding?
2. What is my goal? Exactly what do I want to accomplish? How will assertive behavior on my part help accomplish it?
3. What would my usual nonassertive behavior be? What would I usually do to avoid asserting myself in this situation?
4. Why be assertive? Why would I want to give that up and assert myself instead?
5. What are the blocks I'm experiencing?
   a. Am I holding on to irrational beliefs? If so, what are they?
   b. How can I replace these irrational beliefs with rational ones?
   c. Have I been taught to behave in ways that make it difficult for me to act assertively in the present situation? In what ways? How can I overcome this problem?
   d. What are my rights in this situation? Are these rights worth the effort for me to change my behavior?
6. Am I anxious about asserting myself? What techniques can I use to reduce my anxiety?
7. Have I done my homework? Do I have the information I need to go ahead and act?
8. Can I:
   a. Let the other person know I hear and understand him?
   b. Let the other person know how I feel? What the situation requires?
   c. Tell him what I want? (pp. 175–176)

Finding and Becoming a Role Model

Although actively seeking assertive role models may be a new experience for you, it is one of the best promoters of assertive behavior. A role model is a person whose behaviors, personal style, and specific attributes are emulated by others (Shapiro, Haseltine, and Row, 1978). While different versions of role modeling have been well developed and are very effective in other, predominately male professions, experience has shown that nurses generally do not pursue or emulate professional role models. The lack of emphasis of this notion may be an extension of nurses' limited self-esteem as individuals and as a profession.

As you become more assertive, you probably will start to identify similar behaviors in your friends and colleagues. You can build support for your own assertive attempts by acknowledging and bolstering their behavior as well as by actually visualizing how they might deal with a situation that you are about to encounter. How might you go about finding role models? The most logical beginning is your place of employment. As you begin to notice how people make requests and deal with problems, you may find many assertive superiors, colleagues, and subordinates. Other sources of assertive nurse role models may include nurses in your neighborhood, school system, or volunteer organizations. Another way to locate assertive role models is to attend the presentations of nurse leaders and, if possible, to make a point of meeting them personally. Many nursing leaders are competent, self-confident professionals who can foster your pride in the nursing profession.

In addition to seeking out positive assertive experiences systematically, you may also want to evaluate many of your existing relationships to determine how much energy you are devoting to them and what you are receiving in return. Do you find yourself in negative, draining relationships that you continue because you have known the people "for years"? Remember that assertive nurses are in control of their lives and consciously choose which relationships to continue and which to terminate or to treat as less important. Be assertive and take charge of your time, your life, and your relationships!

As you develop assertive interpersonal skills, you can serve as a role model for others. When your colleagues or subordinates observe you communicating in an assertive manner, you may be just the impetus they need to become assertive. In addition to your stimulating them to be assertive, their presence can be a support to you. For instance, perhaps you want to speak to your head nurse about how frequently you are pulled to another unit on the evening shift. While being sensitive to the risk of seeming to intimidate her with numbers, you still may choose to invite a co-worker with a similar complaint to accompany you. By inviting your co-worker, you are both serving as an assertive role model for her and building-in support for yourself in that she can validate your complaint. Capitalizing on the role model and support aspects of the process while working toward the goal of a more consistent unit assignment certainly focuses on the positive aspects of the issue.

Focusing on the Positive

Being aware of the promoters of assertiveness and using the various skill-building techniques described can be helpful, but you also must acknowledge the impact of your own mental attitude and your environment. Almost everyone functions best in positive surroundings. While assertive behavior can be an effective way of dealing with the problematic areas of your personal and professional life, the essence of assertive behavior is to focus on the positive, thereby preventing some potential problems and offsetting negativism.

While recognizing that many of nurses' current dilemmas are related to the fact that nursing is predominately a female profession, you need to focus on the positive aspects of your female identity. It is time to start feeling good about who you are and what you do. You can begin by looking within yourself and focusing on your personal strengths. What kind of things do you do well? What are some of your positive accomplishments? Think about your past successes. How might you build on them to accomplish future goals?

In your work setting, see to it that you are recognized for your competencies and assertively take credit for your ideas. If you feel stagnant in your job, interview for another position. Whether you actually choose to leave your current position, exploring other possibilities can be a source of stimulation for you.

You can also make an effort to concentrate on the positive aspects of your work and create a more productive work climate. During the course of a normal day, you probably have numerous opportunities to do this. How frequently do you find yourself listening to the same old complaints or commiserating with co-workers in negative gripe sessions? You could be assertive with a complaining co-worker by first clarifying what she wants from you. Does she want you only to listen, or does she want some concrete suggestions? As an example, if the latter is indicated and the complaint centers around a third person's incessant chatter, you could respond in the following way.

DESCRIPTION OF SITUATION AND FEELINGS	"Barb's chatter seems to bug you. I feel that by continuing to listen, you're giving her the message that her behavior is O.K.
EXPECTATIONS	You could try telling her that you have a lot of charting to do and need forty-five minutes of quiet, uninterrupted time.
POSITIVE CONSEQUENCES	If you assert yourself with her about your charting time, you may feel better about the other times when you choose to listen."

By taking such an approach, your thrust is twofold. You change the format from one of negative complaint to positive action, and you get your co-worker actively involved in the process.

To develop this process further, look around any setting and ask yourself, "How can I make this a worthwhile experience? What can I say or do that will bring about learning and fulfillment for me?" You can have this kind of attitude if you decide that you want it, and if you stop allowing yourself to be victimized by yourself or those around you. Learn to reshape things, even adversity, to your advantage by maintaining a positive attitude. Look for the options and opportunities in a situation. For example, when you have an unpleasant task to do, try to convert it into a positive accomplishment. Ask yourself:

- What can I do to make boring staff meetings more interesting?
- How can I tell my co-worker about her body odor in a positive way?
- What can I do to make firing an employee a learning experience?

While it is recognized that not all experiences in life are positive and that sorrow and discomfort need to be experienced so as not to deny reality, many times we permit ourselves to become victims of our own negativity unnecessarily. Instead, as a nurse, you need to make a concentrated effort to acknowledge not only your individual strengths but also those of your nursing colleagues. This kind of positive feedback will provide a means of combating the negative self-image that exists within the nursing profession. Along this line, it is essential to pursue ways of enhancing the confidence of individual nurses inasmuch as the profession's advancement is related to the advancement and success of its individual members. One way this goal can be accomplished is by the authentic use of compliments.

Giving and Receiving Compliments Assertively

Many women are given the message early in life that it is not acceptable to be proud of their accomplishments or that it is not proper to accept compliments in a reinforcing manner. Thus, women find it especially difficult to accept a compliment assertively. Typically, women tend to diminish or negate compliments by making downgrading statements like, "This dress? Oh, I got it on sale ..." or "This suit? Oh, I've had it for years." The implication is that no one else wanted the outfit, that it is not worth much, or that it is outdated.

Generally, little girls are taught to be humble when praised. While boys are expected to boast, it is considered "improper" or "unladylike" for girls to praise themselves. Women are supposed to be embarrassed by flattery. Observe the difference in the way men and women accept compliments. When John is complimented on his golf game, he is likely to respond with "Thanks, wasn't that shot on the fifteenth hole marvelous!" Mary might respond to this same praise with "Oh, well, I've had several lessons."

When you become embarrassed and respond sheepishly to a sincere compliment, the initiator often feels uncomfortable also and is not encouraged to compliment you again. Discounting the compliment gives two messages:

1. It conveys to the person giving the compliment that he did not use good judgment by initiating it. When you discount the compliment, you are saying that you do not value the initiator's opinion. In reality, most of us frequently do value what others think or say and, therefore, should not be too quick to discount a sincere compliment.

2. It conveys that as the recipient, you are not worthy of the compliment. This message is reflective of the recipient's low self-esteem. Accepting a compliment assertively can help to increase your self-esteem.

You can alter these two negative messages by accepting a sincere compliment with either a simple, assertive "thank you" or, better yet, with reinforcement of the compliment. The principle of receiving a sincere compliment assertively is not to discount yourself or the other person, but for both of you to feel good about the compliment. As an example, consider the following hypothetical compliment and its accompanying assertive response.

COMPLIMENT	"You sure are a good nurse!"
ASSERTIVE RESPONSE	"Thank you. I enjoy my work, and it must show."

Even if you do not agree with the compliment, you can still accept it assertively:

COMPLIMENT   "You look great with your hair
                           fixed like that."
ASSERTIVE RESPONSE   "Thank you for noticing."

Similar principles apply to giving compliments assertively. Because assertive behavior is honest, compliments should be genuine. Many feminists believe that women do not naturally give each other praise because a sense of competitiveness for male attention has been promoted among women. In hospital settings, nurses often look to the medical staff for recognition rather than to nursing administration, patients, or each other. Unconsciously, nurses may be competing with each other for recognition and, consequently, not giving each other credit for achievements.

Giving sincere compliments to others can increase their self-esteem and encourage them to be assertive. For example, suppose that you sit on an interdisciplinary committee which has been chaired historically by a male and never by a nurse. A nurse colleague who also sits on the committee is a competent woman who did an outstanding job heading a subcommittee task force. You could promote her appointment as chairperson by recommending that the committee acknowledge her outstanding work with a letter of commendation and see that the chief executive officer, who appoints the committee's chairperson, receives a copy.

When you give a compliment, it is sensible to consider how the recipient feels about compliments. Despite admitted personal discomfort with praise, too often we readily assume that others will be flattered by a compliment. Some individuals find it very difficult to cope with compliments, so difficult that their responses become aggressive. One class participant, a nursing supervisor, described an aide's response in such an instance.

City hospital was making an effort to reward employees for outstanding job performance as identified by patients or their families. When the public relations department received a compliment about an employee, the department issued a letter of commendation. It was the practice of the nursing department for the nursing supervisor to present the letter to the employee personally. In this particular case, when the aide was presented with the letter in front of her peers, she was embarrassed and became overly indignant and flustered. Ultimately, she tore up the letter, threw it in the wastebasket, and stated that her work should not have been singled out because good patient care was the responsibility of all staff on that unit. The nursing supervisor was shocked, hurt, and angry at the response. This recipient's behavior, perceived as ingratitude, was unacceptable to the supervisor.

Although the aide's response was atypical and quite different from how the supervisor herself may have handled the situation had she been the recipient of the compliment, the supervisor came to understand that the subordinate's reaction probably was related to her sense of self-worth. Furthermore, the aide had the right to do whatever she wanted with the letter but also to be responsible for the consequences of her behavior. Needless to say, the incident sensitized the nursing supervisor to the variety of ways people accept compliments. In the future, she will be better prepared for different possible responses to compliments.

The Promoters Can Work for You

Learning to give and accept compliments in an assertive manner usually evolves over a period of months or years and requires attention and practice. For most people, assertive behavior does not "just happen." It is a skill that must be developed and enhanced.

Make a commitment to pursue the promoters of assertive behavior. Of the various promoters available, which have you already mastered? Which will you now consider? We have provided you with several different options. You can decide which will be beneficial for you and then proceed to use them to develop your assertive skills. Allowing the promoters to work for you can lead to a satisfying assertive life-style.

References

Bloom, Lynn, Karen Coburn, and Joan Pearlman. *The New Assertive Woman.* New York: Dell, 1975.

Bolles, Richard Nelson. *What Color Is Your Parachute?* Berkeley, Calif.: Ten Speed Press, 1972.

Bower, Sharon, and Gordon Bower. *Asserting Yourself.* New York: Addison-Wesley, 1976.

Foxworth, Jo. *Wising Up: The Mistakes Women Make in Business and How to Avoid Them.* New York: Delacorte Press, 1980.

Shapiro, Eileen C., Florence P. Haseltine, and Mary P. Row. Moving Up: Role Models, Mentors and the 'Patron System'. *Sloan Management Review* 19 (1978):51–58.

Smith, Manuel. *When I Say No, I Feel Guilty.* New York: Dial Press, 1975.

7
Using Assertive Skills
to Implement Change

Are you satisfied with the way your nursing career is progressing? Is your work setting helping you to meet your career goals? Is your place of employment operating in such a way that you can honestly say you are proud to be a part of it? Are there any changes you would like to see take place in your work setting in order to improve the quality of patient care? If so, what can you do actively and assertively to help bring these things about?

If you are feeling dissatisfied or frustrated in any of these areas, the sense of frustration and discomfort can be used positively as a motivating force to help you implement change. Because human beings are not static, but in dynamic motion through the life cycle, the opportunity to initiate change is an ever-present one. Of course, the stronger your value system and the firmer your commitment to action, the more vigorous the momentum will be to accomplish the desired change.

The focus of the previous chapters has been on helping you to examine the various factors involved in choosing and developing assertive skills for the purpose of changing your individual behavior. Clearly, becoming an assertive person is a process of change. In this chapter, you can examine some ways of using your assertive skills to accomplish broader goals such as changing the setting in which you work and developing support systems.

The nurse who wants to function specifically as a change agent (a designated person from within the setting or someone from the outside whose primary job is to help an organization change) should possess assertive skills. In addition, she should have an understanding of systems and organizational theories, knowledge and experience in the specific area she would like to change, and an understanding of change and the process necessary to implement it.

While it is not within the scope of this book to discuss the variables in an organization that contribute to its complexity, it is recommended that you consult other references on the subject. Because every nurse has the potential to be affected by change and to use assertive skills to initiate it, this chapter includes a discussion of change and how it can be used to benefit patient care as well as nurses and nursing.

What Is Change?

The process which leads to alterations in individual or institutional patterns of behavior is called "change" (Brooten, Hayman, and Naylor, 1978). Change can occur within or between individuals as well as within or between broader systems such as families, organizations, and communities.

The impetus for change varies with individuals. Some people look forward to something new and welcome a change. Others resist change and find security in clinging to what is familiar. Still others are not particularly resistive but are more tolerant and accepting of dissatisfaction so that their need to change is not as great. Then there are those individuals who are so apathetic that they merely accept in a routinized way whatever is imposed upon them, with no apparent desire at all to change either themselves or the systems in which they function.

Frequently, women and nurses become the recipients of change that is initiated and imposed by others. Sometimes these "others" are family members, administrators, physicians, or other colleagues. Traditionally, nurses have been passive in their responses to change and have permitted others to dominate them regardless of the anger or frustrations they may have felt. They have withdrawn from change many times by developing a wait-and-see attitude or by convincing themselves that they had no alternative other than to accept the imposed changes as inevitable. Other times they have reacted aggressively, either by openly resisting the imposed changes or, more often than not, by playing the games of passive resistance or sabotage (described in Chapter 1).

Historically, nurses have been given messages to operate in this manner. Society has fostered "female dependency," while health care agencies, reflecting the broader environment and superimposing essentially male hierarchies, have fostered "nurse dependency."

Clearly, nurses have reacted and responded to change in many different ways, but they have done little to initiate it assertively themselves. By not taking the initiative and becoming actively, assertively involved in the change process, nurses have allowed others to guide and direct their lives.

Change that occurs in this way, without one's active involvement, is change by drift. Brooten, Hayman, and Naylor (1978) describe this kind of change as occurring almost by happenstance, when change accumulates around us, sometimes almost without our noticing. Johnson (1977) refers to this type of change as "unplanned." According to her, most of the change that takes place is unplanned and is a process by which people *react* to their environment. "Planned" change, on the other hand, occurs when people *act* in a predetermined, purposeful, and deliberate way.

Recognizing Change as a Benefit

Contrary to assertive nurses who are open to growth and who change by looking for creativity in themselves and others, many nurses stifle change because they feel threatened. Feelings of threat make them cling to their defenses and remain reluctant to take risks. To bring about change, nurses must be willing to modify old behaviors, develop new skills, and stop permitting themselves to be victims of their environment.

How frequently have you heard yourself or other nurses say, "Oh, we can't do that . . . It's never been done . . . The supervisor wouldn't go for it . . ." or "We'd better ask Dr. Jones first. . . ." Such comments are often unnecessary. More gains and advancements could be made if nurses would take the individual initiative to implement change, particularly in their work settings, without automatically and unnecessarily asking permission first. Of course, they must be initially knowledgeable, well prepared, alert to the risks involved, and aware of possible consequences. Also, they have a responsibility to inform the appropriate people about their actions. But there is a difference between informing others and asking their permission.

Granted, there are occasions when it is appropriate for permission to be requested. Organizational goals need to be considered, and many times it is essential to obtain approval in order to proceed. Besides, superiors can lend their guidance and support, thus contributing to a smooth transition and the sound implementation of change. Additionally, because the authority figure has the ultimate responsibility for events in the setting, that individual has a right to be informed, to be involved, and to sanction or veto the proposals of employees. Yet, all too often, nurses neglect making progress because they think that each and every detail of their nursing practice needs to be checked out with the authority. Instead, nurses must take an assertive step forward and risk.

Although traditionally nurses have been encouraged to operate from a dependent, submissive position, they can "shift gears" and learn to initiate planned change. Nurses need to recognize that in order to advance individually and collectively, it is essential to change from being "apathetic receptors" to becoming "active initiators." Nurses must realize that power and control of the nursing profession begins with power and control of each individual nurse over herself, her own nursing practice, and her own professional career.

Not only is initiating change a responsibility of the individual nurse, but it is also the responsibility of nursing educators and nursing management. Nursing educators, especially those in continuing education, have a role to play in raising nurses' consciousness about issues such as the value of a more vigorous approach to nursing career growth and development, and the importance of making the work environment more conducive to the advancement of nurses and nursing. Obviously, nursing educators must provide skill development for individual nurses to pursue such changes.

Likewise, nursing managers have a responsibility for initiating change. They can improve the work environment by initiating changes themselves, by supporting other nurses in making positive changes, and by facilitating the career development of nurses within their settings. While it is recognized that the primary role of most health care organizations is patient care, the fact remains that many nursing managers within health care organizations need to find ways of loosening organizational structures, rules, and procedures to enable more nurses to move through the various career stages so essential for career development. Often, organizational policies and traditions are too restrictive to permit such development (Dalton, Thompson, and Price, 1977).

Because the environment has a significant influence on the successful implementation of change, it is necessary to examine the environment in which you practice. The assertive nurse identifies the type of work setting that will promote her career growth and considers this as one of the criteria in selecting a place of employment. When interviewing, she becomes actively involved in the process by asking questions of the prospective employer to determine whether the environment and opportunities available meet her expectations. Once she acquires a position, she monitors whether staying in that setting will promote the attainment of her identified career goals.

When is the last time you critically examined your work setting in this respect? How does your work environment contribute to your growth and development? Is your individual creativity being enhanced? Do your job description and title reflect the work you do? If not, why not? What about the amount of responsibility and authority you have? Are they comparable with what you want and feel you deserve?

While maintaining loyalty and responsibility to the job, do not permit yourself to be a victim of the institution in which you work. Periodically determine how much of your time is being devoted in a self-sacrificing way for the job or institution. Assertively assess if that is really what you want for yourself. If not, change your priorities. Evaluate whether you are being asked to sacrifice beyond the time or effort you are paid for. Ask yourself if your salary reflects the quality of the job you do. If not, why not? Has the thought occurred to you that remaining nonassertive may be costing you money?

Make a commitment to use your assertive skills to change creatively some of the inequities you have identified. In order to do this in an effective way, knowledge of the process of planned change is necessary. Just as there are varying degrees of assertiveness, there are varying degrees of involvement in the change process. The assertive nurse determines for herself how involved in this process she wants to become and how she will manage her involvement.

Using the Process of Planned Change to Change the Work Setting Assertively

Although many theoretical models describe the change process in organizations, the problem-solving model used by Brooten, Hayman, and Naylor (1978) as an approach to planned change is presented here because of its effectiveness and familiarity to nurses as a basis for the nursing process. The stages of *assessment, planning, implementation,* and *evaluation* are used as a frame of reference from which to understand the process of planned change. In this approach, there is collaboration at all levels and at each step of the change process, including the reason for the change, definition of the problem, goal setting, strategies for action, and evaluation of the process. No one dictates. Mutual respect is communicated by a distribution of power and purposefulness at the collective level. The process is an open one, and the direction of change is the result of consensus, meaning that general agreement exists among workers regarding the actions to be taken.

This type of involvement may be foreign to some people within the organization, who from past experience have learned to prefer having their superiors tell them what to do. Additionally, it can be unsettling to realize that the exact outcome is not predetermined but evolves as the group works together.

The principal advantage of this approach to planned change is that it generates commitment on the part of organizational members. However, change by this route takes a long time to implement; for major organizational change, the time involved may be approximately 2 to 4 years. Thus, a great deal of investment is made in terms of time and energy, but the results are more likely to be satisfying and durable. If carried out properly, the process can have a unifying effect on the system. This model can be used effectively by assertive nurses who are interested in initiating and implementing change.

An example of such a nurse is Sharon, an assertive staff nurse interested in initiating a change in the ambulatory care department at Brickmont Hospital, where she works. Several factors are motivating her to introduce the idea of flexible working hours into her department. The nurses in ambulatory care have always worked 8:00 A.M. to 4:30 P.M., but Sharon feels there would be many advantages to a more flexible schedule. The ambulatory care department is part of a teaching health center and is very busy. Recently, in order to accommodate an increased volume of patients, the medical residents began seeing patients as early as 7:30 A.M. Often these patients leave the clinic without seeing a nurse, thereby missing out on important health teaching and follow-up. Patients are also confused about future appointments.

Because of an increase in the number of operating room cases, the surgical residents gradually started seeing their patients later in the day. Consequently, either the nurses work overtime, or patients do not receive appropriate nursing interventions. The nurses are becoming frustrated by working overtime; they also complain about not having enough time to get organized in the morning before being barraged with requests, and they do not have sufficient time at the end of the day to conclude the shift to their satisfaction.

Because of the gradual extension of patient hours, communication between physicians and nurses has become fragmented and tense. The staff presented the problem to the nursing director of ambulatory care, but the solutions she suggested did not resolve the problems. Although solving them is not Sharon's responsibility, she is affected by the situation and wants to do something about it assertively.

In addition to the work-related factors just mentioned, Sharon's life situation soon will be such that she will not be able to leave her home until 8:30 A.M. Sharon likes many aspects of her job and does not want to leave. She believes that flexible work hours for the nursing staff, which would expand the period of nursing coverage, might address several of the problems identified. She approaches this potential solution knowledgeable about the change process and willing to invest herself in it.

In order to effect change, it is necessary to make a commitment to work and expend energy in order to get what you want. Be willing to invest yourself, and assume responsibility for leading the action in order to accomplish change. For instance, offer to chair a committee or head a task force if that is what it takes to implement your idea.

The nurse who is contemplating the introduction of change in an organization needs to identify the problem accurately, if there is one, in the system that is stimulating the initiation of the change. Confusing the symptoms of the problem with the problem itself can result in the entire change effort focusing on the wrong issue (Spradley, 1980). The importance of an accurate identification of the problem on an organizational level parallels the importance of accurately defining the decision to be made when initiating an assertion on an interpersonal level.

Nurses also need to determine whether the change is actually necessary. While purposeful, planned change can have positive effects and is often needed, it is justified only if it can provide something better than what already exists. Too often change is initiated merely for its own sake or as a means of keeping up with a current trend instead of for substantial reasons.

In the situation in the ambulatory care department at Brickmont, Sharon believes that her reasons for initiating change have merit. With her new proposal of "flextime," not only would patients receive more comprehensive care, but the nurses and physicians should be better satisfied and, hopefully, able to work together more effectively.

The ramifications of changes that nurses initiate, especially with regard to the overall organizational system, are influenced by the type of facility in which they practice, by the amount of support they receive from their superiors, and by the positions they hold in the organization. For instance, changes initiated by an assertive staff nurse are likely to be confined to the immediate area in which she works, although they may have broader implications.

In Sharon's case, she plans to call attention to an inefficient scheduling routine, suggest something better in its place, and help in the implementation of the change within the confines of the ambulatory care department. However, if her flextime suggestion is successful, it may be implemented in other departments and eventually be integrated throughout the facility.

Change can occur on a small scale on an individual unit between nurses, co-workers, patients, superiors, and subordinates. It can also occur on a large scale within whole departments or throughout an entire organization.

Assessing the Environment

When change in an organization is necessary and appropriate, the assertive nurse who is initiating it needs to consider various factors that will influence the success or failure of her change efforts. Among them is an assessment of the environment. This includes determining the *interest and motivation* for change, the *potential resistances* that may impede the change process, and the nature of the *existing power bases*. When first assessing a system or any of its component parts, such as the particular nursing area in which she would like to institute change, the assertive nurse needs to recognize that the nursing unit in which she works affects and is affected by all the other parts of the organization. It does not operate in isolation but has a relationship to all other aspects of the organization.

For instance, Sharon would be wise to consider and plan how the initiation of flextime for the nursing staff in the ambulatory care department will affect coordination with other departments such as the scheduling clerks, x-ray, the pharmacy, and the laboratory. Also, she should consider specific implications it might have regarding patients, staff supervision, communication with other agency personnel, meetings, or staff development programs. Even small details like staff transportation to and from work, the availability of parking facilities, and bus schedules need to be considered.

The assertive nurse wanting to implement a change also must consider how much dissatisfaction exists in the present situation and how committed people are to positive action. Typically, people complain about what they do not like, but they are not seriously interested in doing anything in a positive, assertive way to effect change. The most durable and beneficial changes occur when individuals within the system are interested and motivated to accept a share of the responsibility and are willing to invest in bringing about the change. People are more likely to assume responsibility if there is a large gap between what they want and what exists, particularly if the desired change will satisfy their needs for achievement, interpersonal relationships, or recognition (Hertzberg, 1969).

In this regard, Sharon needs to determine if the rest of the nursing staff in the ambulatory care area are willing to join her in her efforts to improve the situation. How unhappy are they? Are they interested in investing time and energy into trying tentative solutions? How committed is the staff to assuring quality patient care?

Change is easier to implement in a conducive environment. If the environment is not favorable, though, work can be done to improve it. When the individuals within an organization are blindly committed to the organization or when they feel alienated, the climate for change is weak. On the contrary, if the work setting is viewed by the individual as an avenue for personal or professional growth, an ideal relationship is likely to exist between organizational and personal goals. An atmosphere in which the problems are challenging and people feel personally secure probably is the best climate for change (Brooten, Hayman, and Naylor, 1978). Such an atmosphere promotes assertiveness among employees. Mutual respect exists between employer and employees, with each being aware of the other's expectations through open, honest, and direct communication.

Conflict and resistance are natural parts of the change process. Their presence should come as no suprise to the nurse who is knowledgeable about the process of change. In fact, forces that both promote and resist change probably coexist. Kurt Lewin suggests that the presence of these opposing forces keeps the system in balance (Benne and Birnbaum, 1969). Change upsets this balance (or "homeostasis"). Therefore, the assertive nurse who wants to bring about change either must increase the forces promoting change, decrease the forces resisting change, or both (Spradley, 1980). Comparing the relative strengths of these two forces can help you to decide on appropriate strategies for action (Brooten, Hayman, and Naylor, 1978).

In the ambulatory care setting at Brickmont, Sharon has identified several forces that would promote the change to flexible work hours. Patients and physicians most likely would support flextime because it would mean better, more efficient service. Some of the staff would like the idea of having a choice about work hours. Joan, one of the three head nurses, is very patient centered and could be counted on to support a change that would benefit patients. A second head nurse, Lucille, is very energetic and flexible. She probably would support the change also, especially if she believed that it would improve the work environment and if her staff really wanted it. The nursing director has been receptive to trying innovative solutions as long as they were well planned. On the other hand, the resistive forces most likely would include a third head nurse, Josephine, who is rigid but well organized. Undoubtedly, she would view flextime as a complication to the management of her unit. In the past, this head nurse has been skeptical of any change with the potential of upsetting her system. The payroll and personnel departments also might be resistive since a change of this type would require adjustments from them.

When initiating change, it is also important to assess the sources and styles of power used by individuals or groups within the organization. People may acquire power from many sources, such as their designated positions, control, knowledge, skill, relationships, connections, and tenure. An understanding of who holds power and how that power is used is crucial to a successful, assertive implementation of change. Being aware of the power bases in your setting will be advantageous when planning strategies for the implementation of change later on.

Sharon assessed the relative strength of the power bases of the probable promoters and resisters of the flextime idea. The ambulatory care nursing director and physicians have fairly strong power bases, while the personnel and payroll departments have minimal power in this organization. On analysis, Sharon was surprised at the amount of power she estimated to be wielded by Josephine, the rigid head nurse. This head nurse had long-standing, fiercely loyal relationships with several influential physicians. Although this head nurse might not be able to exercise enough power to block the project totally, she could make implementation very difficult.

Various means of exercising power can be employed. Some powerful individuals may operate by purposefully preventing con-

flict from surfacing by communicating that devastating consequences will result if there is not strict adherence to certain rules
and regulations. Others withhold essential information or deliber-
ately create a crisis, discontent, or dissension as power tactics. For
example, the potentially resistive head nurse could withhold essential information about vacations, layoffs, or sick leave to
sabotage the project.

Planning the Change

Just as planning is an important step in the process of executing a
given assertion, it is crucial in implementing change. In this step,
the groundwork for action is laid. The successful implementation of
change is dependent upon quality planning that is well developed
and comprehensive. In this stage of the change process, consideration must be given to the establishment of *support,* the *identification of goals,* and the development of *strategies for action,* including *ways of dealing with resistance.*

The assertive nurse knows that her chances of implementing
change successfully will be greater if she can convince others of the
value of her idea and elicit their support effectively. Consequently,
the formation and development of a support group is essential.
The support group can provide strength to the change process by
supplying numbers of people, varied skills, credibility or status,
contacts with other people or groups, or financial support, if needed. It is especially advantageous if members of the group are competent, attractive, articulate, sensitive, and skillful in assertive
communication.

Since implementing change effectively is related to the constructive involvement of the people within the system, it is helpful
to include them early in the change process during the planning
stage. Their ideas, knowledge, and interests should be taken into
account when goals are formed and decisions are made so that a
consensus can be reached. In this way, not only will quality planning result, but a built-in commitment will result on the part of the
group to work toward the success of the effort.

In preparation for the presentation of her idea of flextime to the nursing staff in Brickmont's ambulatory care department, Sharon spoke with her head nurse and the nursing director of that area. They supported her efforts to do something constructive to correct the existing unsatisfactory conditions and gave her encouragement to present her idea to the staff. As a way of planning for the staff meeting where she was to present her idea, Sharon used the Assertive Checklist introduced in Chapter 6:

1. *Clarify the situation and focus on the issue. Listen to what's being said and validate your understanding.*

Sharon accomplished this first step by assessing the environment and determining the interest and readiness of the staff for change.

2. *What is my goal? Exactly what do I want to accomplish? How will assertive behavior on my part help accomplish it?*

Both long- and short-term goals need to be established. The long-term goals should clearly identify the end results desired, while the short-term goals should serve as milestones along the way. The goals need to be realistic, appropriate to the desired change, achievable within a designated period of time, and measurable. Through periodic monitoring during the process of their attainment, modifications can be made if necessary. However, if changes are made, they should be done by the same type of consensus used to formulate the original plan (Brooten, Hayman, and Naylor, 1978).

Sharon's personal goal is to start and finish her work day later. Organizational goals include: (*a*) comparable care for all patients since they would be able to see a nurse regardless of their appointment times, (*b*) a better-paced workday for the staff, and (*c*) more face-to-face contact with the physicians, thereby improving communications. Sharon decided that assertively proposing a change to flextime would help to accomplish these goals.

3. *What would my usual nonassertive behavior be? What*

would I usually do to avoid asserting myself in this situation?

Sharon's usual nonassertive behavior would be to do nothing or to continue to complain and eventually resign from the ambulatory care department to find another job with later hours.

4. *Why be assertive? Why would I want to give that up and assert myself instead?*

By being assertive and proposing a change, Sharon envisions the following advantages:

- She would have an opportunity to participate in a stimulating, innovative project.
- She would be implementing her commitment to quality patient care.
- She would not have to change jobs in order to work later hours.

5. *What are the blocks I'm experiencing?*

   a. Am I holding on to irrational beliefs? If so, what are they?

   b. How can I replace these irrational beliefs with rational ones?

Sharon identified certain irrational beliefs along with their corresponding rational counterparts. In this way, she can compare irrational fears with rational risks.

IRRATIONAL BELIEF	My colleagues won't like the idea of flextime.
RATIONAL COUNTERPART	Some of them may be in a similar personal situation and would welcome the opportunity to choose another starting time.

IRRATIONAL BELIEF	Flextime is too complex to implement.
RATIONAL COUNTERPART	We have good management in this department. They are capable of implementing the concept and would be challenged by such a project.
IRRATIONAL BELIEF	The patients will be confused by the nurses' hours. They will dislike the idea.
RATIONAL COUNTERPART	The patients may be very willing to tolerate different schedules if they are assured that a nurse will see them regardless of their appointment times.

c. *Have I been taught to behave in ways that make it difficult for me to act assertively in the present situation? In what ways? How can I overcome this problem?*

Sharon has thought about her background and acknowledges that she has been taught that "good girls are seen and not heard." In the past, she has not been rewarded for being outspoken and assertive. Consequently, it is hard for her muster the courage to speak up and suggest a change. She tries to overcome this problem by identifying the advantages of being assertive and by focusing on her personal rights.

d. *What are my rights in this situation? Are these rights worth the effort for me to change my behavior?*

Sharon determined that the following rights were worth the effort to propose flextime assertively:

- The right to ask for a change in the work system
- The right to express an opinion

- The right to define quality nursing care
- The right to provide that care
- The right of patients to receive safe, quality care

6. *Am I anxious about asserting myself? What techniques can I use to reduce my anxiety?*

Sharon was anxious about suggesting the flextime idea at the next staff meeting. So during her lunch hour preceding the meeting, she took a brisk walk to dissipate some of the tension physically. She also practiced some deep-breathing techniques and rehearsed what she would say.

7. *Have I done my homework? Do I have the information I need to go ahead and act?*

Sharon had read most of the information currently available on flextime and had talked with people who work in other organizations where various approaches to flexible work hours were in effect. When presenting her suggestions, she decided to keep in mind the following general principles (Brooten, Hayman, and Naylor, 1978):

- Present the rationale for the change based on accurate data and solid facts
- Focus discussion on the issues that are necessary for accomplishing the change and those that are the most meaningful
- Emphasize *goals,* not roles; *collaboration,* not competition; and *ideas,* not personalities
- Identify the proposed consequences of the change as specifically and concretely as possible
- Use language that is easily understood and familiar to everyone involved

8. *Can I:*

a. *Let the other person know I hear and understand him?*
b. *Let the other person know how I feel?*
c. *Tell him what I want? What the situation requires?*

Sharon made arrangements in advance of the staff meeting to have her ideas of flextime placed on the agenda. Also, she made sure that there was sufficient time for her presentation. She went to the staff meeting and initiated the proposed change by using her knowledge of assertive communication skills. In an assertive manner, she said:

EMPATHIC COMPONENT	"I realize that all of us are busy and that new ideas take time.
DESCRIPTION OF FEELINGS AND SITUATION	But I'm feeling overwhelmed with the work pace and discouraged that we [nurses] are not seeing some of the patients. Besides, I will have to begin working later hours soon.
EXPECTATIONS	I think flexible work hours can help several of these situations. I would like to see us implement a well-planned change to some version of flextime. I have gathered a lot of information about it and want to present it to you for your consideration."

Sharon was pleased that most of the management and staff were receptive, even enthusiastic, about her suggestion. However, because of the numerous variables involved, she knew that change would not occur overnight.

When contemplating change, it is best to plan it in stages and to allow sufficient time for it to be assimilated. In addition, there will be less resistance to change if some "anchor points" are maintained by keeping certain aspects of the environment stable and constant instead of introducing too many changes at once.

Besides establishing support and identifying goals, which are important steps in planning, it is also necessary to develop strategies for action during this stage. In developing strategies for action, particular attention should be paid to the established goals. Goals may be thought of as "what" is to be done, while strategies are "how" they will be attained. The selection of strategies should be based on the information obtained during the previous assessment stage. In addition, when deciding on a plan of action, it is wise to include an alternative plan in case the first one fails.

Schaller (1972) suggests four general strategies for implementing change: coercion, cooptation, conflict or confrontation, and cooperation.

Coercion, which means forcing change on people through the use of authority or power, can take several forms. For example, the director of nursing in the ambulatory care department at Brickmont could have decided to implement the change to flextime by autocratically diagnosing the problem, setting goals, and determining strategies for action. She could have called in certain subordinates to discuss the situation but still have guided the direction of the change authoritatively.

The main advantage of this strategy is having some deliberate direction to the change, but the main disadvantage is that it represents less than full coordination of efforts. The result is that different people may attempt to change the organization in different directions.

In another form of coercion, the same director of nursing could have decided to impose the change to flextime solely by a written announcement, without any type of interaction with the employees. While this form of coercion may be logical, it tends to be merely a paper-and-pencil creation that employees in their day-to-day work roles do not enact, since the person making the decision is not the one involved in the daily execution of it.

While change by coercion may be necessary in some cases, generally it tends to create resentment and frustration among employees as well as a discrepancy between what is imposed and what is enacted.

Cooptation occurs when the opposition is brought into the

support group for the purpose of compromising or bargaining. Something is usually given up at the same time that something else is gained. This can result in a weakening of the forces in that the group not only becomes more diverse but the move is also perceived as "buying off" the enemy.

An illustration of this strategy, using the flextime example, might be to offer Josephine, the resistant head nurse, extra staff for her area if she would be willing to go along with the new proposal. While accomplishing a consistency in scheduling arrangements, this strategy probably would cause divisiveness and dissension among the other head nurses who would not receive a comparable benefit of an increase in staff.

Conflict or confrontation, when introduced purposefully in a constructive manner, may serve to clarify the issues involved; if used destructively, it can have a divisive effect and impede change by perpetuating resistances that already exist. If Josephine, the head nurse who opposed the idea of flextime, were confronted in a positive way, most likely she would respond favorably. However, if she were confronted in a negative manner about her rigid, controlling behavior, probably she would retaliate by increasing her resistance and creating additional barriers to the implementation of the proposed change.

Cooperation, which occurs when individuals within the system are collaborating, is the most widely used approach to planned change. Although it may be time consuming, its effects are likely to be durable. Once Sharon enlisted the support of her boss and coworkers, a cooperative effort evolved. A series of planning meetings was held to identify strategies for action.

Specific change strategies have to be planned on an individual basis within each setting. When planning strategies, it is advisable to hold brainstorming sessions to examine several possibilities. However, one overall, clear, well-defined course of action should be chosen in order to avoid confusion and unnecessary expenditures of energy and resources in different directions. The enactment of several solutions can cause confusion and lead to failure (Spradley, 1980).

Failure of the change effort also can result if ample consideration is not given to planning specific strategies to deal with previously identified or potential sources of resistance. Chances are that the people who will resist change the most will be those who are insecure, who have invested a lot of themselves in the current operation, who see no personal benefit to the change, who view it as opposition to their value systems, or who see it as a threat to their comfort.

A potentially effective way of dealing with resistance is to show how the proposed change will benefit the resister by the enhancement of personal values or goals. Another way is to be sensitive and receptive to the ideas of the people affected by the change and to involve them early in the planning process so that they will have a personal investment in the change. They will be less likely to be resistive if your method and leadership style meet with their approval, if they like you, and if their self-esteem is protected.

During the planning sessions at Brickmont, which included representatives from all levels of the ambulatory care nursing department, the values of Josephine (the head nurse who was identified as a potential resister) were kept in mind. Since she valued consistency and control, one of the change strategies was to plan around her as a stable variable. Thus, when the group discussed supervisory coverage, it was suggested that the other two head nurses initially work the earlier and later shifts, leaving Josephine free to keep her usual hours for awhile. Also, for Josephine's benefit, it was clarified that the head nurses could have the freedom to set up the details of flextime in whatever manner would work best for them. In this way, they would be assured some control of their staff, who might be starting work earlier or leaving later than they would. The group was perceptive enough to recognize Josephine's ability to organize so they readily supported Sharon's suggestion to involve Josephine directly in the change process by asking her to help develop various schedules for their consideration at a later date. The group decided that the best time to implement flextime would be in the fall after most of the staff vacations had been completed.

The best-laid plans may go astray if ample consideration is not given to the timing of the initiation of change. Just as it is crucial to the implementation of an individual assertion, timing is important to the assertive implementation of organizational change.

The director of nursing in the ambulatory care department at Brickmont recognized the advantage of implementing Sharon's idea of flextime at a time when the staff was interested in a change and when she had someone like Sharon to promote it enthusiastically. Taking advantage of the opportunity to initiate change in an area at a time when the leadership is strong and committed to the new idea is sound, strategic planning.

Implementing the Change

While the major tasks involved in the assessment and planning phases of the change process are completed before the actual implementation stage begins, the competent, assertive change agent realizes that continued assessment is beneficial. By monitoring the change while it is being implemented, adjustments and modifications can be made if the need arises. Problems may surface that were not anticipated earlier, so adaptability and flexibility during this stage are essential.

As implied previously in the discussion of "timing," it is wise to begin enacting the change in an area where success will be achieved so that credence will be given to the new idea. Beginning the change in a limited area, such as a carefully selected nursing unit like the ambulatory care department, on a trial basis can be a desirable mechanism of introduction. It can also supply data as a means of evaluating the process and the final outcomes of the project.

Since honesty and trust are essential to the successful attainment of change, the exact intentions behind initiating a "trial run" should be stated assertively. Although this does not apply in Sharon's case, in other facilities when change is going to be widespread after its introduction in a selected area, that message should be given clearly to all concerned. People must not be led to believe that the change is simply "experimental" and that their feedback will be considered before implementing the change in other areas if, in reality, a decision to the contrary has already been made. Instead, such a message could be communicated accurately by letting people know that the change will expand to the facility as a whole, that a given unit has been selected to introduce it, and that the feedback received from personnel will have an influence on the *way* the change is implemented elsewhere.

Throughout the various phases of the change process, open, honest, and direct communication (assertiveness) is crucial. To the extent possible, everyone involved must know what is happening, why it is happening, and what specifically is expected of them. To monitor the process actively and ensure continuity, especially if the change is a major one, someone should work on the change daily. In addition, people need to receive rewards and recognition for their efforts. Implementing change is a demanding task, although it can also be challenging and rewarding. Helping people to recognize that their efforts are appreciated and valued is an important part of sustaining the momentum and motivation for change (Brooten, Hayman, and Naylor, 1978).

At Brickmont, the director of nursing in the ambulatory care department helped to supply additional impetus to the initiation of flextime by providing the group with resource materials and positive suggestions for implementation. Furthermore, she praised their efforts to nursing management from the inpatient area, who in turn invited them to present the idea at a staff development program. Once flextime was introduced, a comparison was made between the number of absences taken before and after its initiation. The favorable results reinforced the staff's decision to continue the change effort.

Evaluating the Process

Beginning the evaluation process during the implementation stage of the change is a way of helping to maintain motivation. By pausing periodically to evaluate the progress that has been made, people can recognize their accomplishments in a tangible way. Progress should be measured against preestablished goals and a timetable. During these evaluation periods, questions should be asked regarding whether the group is accomplishing what it set out to do originally and, if not, why not.

A realistic evaluation of the change process and its progress must be done, with modifications made in the strategies if necessary. Data acquired as a result of an evaluation of the completed project will supply valuable insights for the implementation of future changes as well as identifying areas needing additional planning efforts. The fact that energies are even directed toward an evaluation procedure helps to reinforce the accountability and responsibility aspect of the change process. Accountability and responsibility are just as important to the implementation of change as they are to successful assertions.

Brickmont's outpatient department staff found that flexible working hours solved some of the problems identified. However, it also created a few more. The consensus was that the minimal problems it created were manageable and the benefits of the concept far outweighed the disadvantages. The staff was further motivated to work on other aspects of the identified problem which flextime could not solve. The implementation of flextime into Brickmont's outpatient department system was monitored closely until it became an integral part of the daily operation.

Follow-up of the change should continue until it is an established part of the system. Once the change is internalized by those affected and it maintains itself autonomously, the change process is completed and stabilized. Measures then should be taken to sustain the change and to "refreeze" the system. Stabilization, an essential part of the change process, solidifies the change and restores balance to the system. While there may still be room for improvement, if the change process as previously described has been optimally effective, the system will be in dynamic equilibrium. Power will be balanced and interdependent. People will have respect for each other, and the system will be open and adaptable—ready to meet the new challenges and changes of the future.

Developing Support Systems to Implement Change and Maintain Assertive Skills

Once you have developed proficient assertive skills and are ready to embark on effecting change, take the time to ask yourself, "How will I maintain my assertive skills during the change process?"

While you are developing assertive skills, you usually have guidance and support from group facilitators and other participants. After the group disbands, however, you can keep the concepts alive by assembling resources and support systems.

To keep assertive concepts keen and readily available, you can refer frequently to the several books and articles on the subject. Inquire if the library in your setting has information on assertiveness and, if not, request it. Arrange for references on the subject to be handy on nursing units since sources of effective interpersonal skills are equally as important as texts on other aspects of nursing. By keeping such information within easy access and by sharing it with your friends and family, you can build an individual support system. Ask others to promote your assertiveness by reminding you when you are behaving either aggressively or passively.

Taking an assertiveness course with a friend or co-worker is another effective way of building in future support. The two of you, or a group, can meet regularly to assess and support each other's progress. By encouraging others to be assertive also, you can help to strengthen and improve family and work relationships. Building a support system sounds easy, yet this idea is not generally well developed within nursing. Frequently, the comment is made that "nurses just don't stick together" (Kelly, 1978). Many nurses blame a lack of cohesiveness on the fact that they are a predominately female profession, while others feel that it is difficult to develop mutual trust necessary for support because there is so much diversity within the nursing profession. Whatever the reason, the time has come for nurses to respect and acknowledge their differences while not focusing on them exclusively. Assertive nurses need to move on to unifying issues and focus on the positive . . . on what is possible.

By focusing more on strengths and commonalities, and less on diversity, nurses can learn to accept differences and work together more effectively. The relationship between accepting the differences of others and giving them support carries over into how nurses perceive and treat colleagues who choose nontraditional work settings or pursue nonnursing endeavors. When referring to these colleagues, many nurses immediately say, "Well, she's left nursing." This shortsighted attitude usually alienates the venturesome colleague who may subsequently be reluctant to acknowledge her nursing background. The more positive approach is to view the person as a nurse-attorney or a nurse-politician, to support her, and to determine how this nurse, working in another arena, can help nursing.

For example, an assertive feminist public health nurse was responsible for developing a rape crisis center. This accomplishment led her to advocacy work for the victims of violent crime, and eventually she ran for public office. The media described her as a dynamic, resourceful former public health nurse. When she approached local nurses for support in her campaign, however, many were hesitant to support her, pointing out that she was not a member of their group and that it had been years since she had practiced nursing. Fortunately, some astute nurses within the group recognized the importance of supporting such a candidate and did so. They could accept her different career path and instead focus on the fact that if she won the election, she would control a large county budget that determined the activities of the local health department. All of this potential influence may have been forfeited if the attitude had prevailed that she was "no longer a nurse."

One way to put aside differences and focus on supporting and promoting one another is to develop a formal support network. Men have always had the "good ole boy network" that provides support in the form of information, contacts, guidance, advice, and protection. Recently, women, especially those in business, have recognized the value of a formal support system and are consciously creating what has been termed "network systems." This involves deliberate, planned (assertive) action to communicate regularly with those people whom you identify as potentially helpful to your personal and career development as well as to the advancement of the profession.

To determine the extent of your support, ask yourself the following questions:

1. Do I interact regularly with my peers and co-workers about general nursing topics rather than specific work-related ones?
2. Do I interact regularly with colleagues who have posi-

tions similar to mine but who practice in other work settings?

3. Does my work setting provide a structure for such interaction?

If there is no current structure in your work setting to promote regular interaction with peers, you may want to request one. Using your assertive skills, you could present the rationale for a staff nurse organization, a supervisory meet-and-discuss group, or a department head council—whatever structure would meet the needs of your group. A positive, mutually supportive work environment can develop. If you look for, request, and organize support, you will receive it. Likewise, you will find yourself supporting others. As a result of actively seeking and receiving support from others, your personal energies and strengths will be reinforced. Outside the work setting, you may want to pursue special interest groups—and, if none exists, develop one!

Kelly (1978) writes about such a support system that she calls a "good new nurse network." Such networks would promote support of nurses, for nurses and create an atmosphere wherein nurses could share, trust, and depend on each other. Small groups of assertive nurses could develop a support system for assertive behavior by creating such networks. Although this kind of networking takes time and energy, the rewards justify the investment. As a result of being part of a network, you will be better informed about activities within your work settings as well as the settings of other nurses. This will enable you to make more effective clinical and career decisions, request and effect appropriate changes, and at times negotiate from a position of strength because of your information.

While nursing should be the primary support system for nurses, it is wise to develop other effective relationships with non-nurse health care providers. Today's patients require such complex care that nurses cannot isolate themselves from nonnursing colleagues. Use your assertive skills to draw on the resources of these co-workers. As an assertive nurse, you will learn how to mesh the strengths of the various health team members toward the ultimate goal of quality patient care.

Another aspect of developing support systems is to elicit help from nursing management. Assertive nurses ask for support specifically instead of just complaining about the lack of it. Nurses in many settings look exclusively to physicians or patients for their rewards and support. You can use your assertive skills, however, to shift this focus by requesting that nursing management also be a source of rewards and support.

For example, when accepting a new job, you may want to be very specific about asking your new boss how she will support you during the critical period when you are learning new job responsibilities and establishing relationships with your subordinates. You can also ask assertively what specific indicators you will receive regarding your progress. One assertive nurse asked her new boss, the director of nursing, for suggestions as to how she, as the new assistant director, could become better acquainted with her subordinates. When presented with such a specific request for support, not only did the director suggest one-to-one luncheons, but she offered to cover the expense! Often nursing management sincerely wants to support individual nurses, although they may not always know how. Be assertive and tell them.

The Importance of Nursing Leadership Support

The degree to which nurses can effect change in health care is to a great extent dependent upon the recognition and acceptance of assertive concepts by individual nurses and nursing leadership, from both the education and practice settings. Although assertiveness is a contemporary term, nursing leaders have been calling for this type of behavior for years. These leaders have been challenging nurses to "throw off the chains of subservience" and to function responsibly, autonomously, and accountably. Nurses have been encouraged to speak out, to exert power, and to stand up for their own rights as well as the rights of patients. When nursing leaders present such expectations, they have a corresponding obligation to promote and endorse the development of skills to meet these challenges. While this call to action has certainly been appropriate, nurse leaders need to acknowledge that nurses do not just become self-confident, accountable, or outspoken; rather, they need help developing in these areas.

Without identifying it as such, many administrators already have assertive expectations of their staff. "Effective interpersonal skills," which include assertiveness, often are included in professional job descriptions. As many nurses find themselves functioning in more complex health care systems, they realize that they need more sophisticated "people skills" in communication and management. If good interpersonal skills are deemed necessary to interact effectively with physicians, co-workers, subordinates, and students, then nurses need to be evaluated in their proficiency in this area and given opportunities to develop or improve these skills. Some administrators feel that effective interpersonal skills are a minimal expectation and that nurses should have developed these skills in school. In reality, many staff nurses and nurse educators, as well as nurses in middle and top management positions, do not have such skills. A definite gap exists between what should be and what is.

Certainly a factor for consideration is whose responsibility it is to assure that nurses possess such skills. While some nurse managers may argue that it is the individual nurse's responsibility to develop such skills, many others believe that because an assertive staff promotes quality patient care, it is management's responsibility to see that the staff are as assertive as possible. Quality patient care often is not provided because nurses are afraid to challenge questionable directives, to insist that a policy is either followed or appropriately overlooked, or to truly act as patient advocates.

The nurse manager in both the educational and practice setting who wants her respective faculty or staff to be more assertive needs to seek opportunities to help her employees recognize that they have behavioral options and then to develop the skills to exercise those options. To that end, nursing leadership can actively promote assertiveness programs provided within the work setting or those sponsored by outside organizations.

When a nurse functions in an assertive manner, can she be assured of support from management? Not always, as the following all-too-frequent example illustrates: When Jill, the evening nurse, came on duty, she heard in report that Mrs. Smith, who had been admitted a few hours ago, was very anxious about the possibility that she might have a serious debilitating disease. Furthermore, Jill was told that the request for Mrs. Smith's test results had been transmitted to the laboratory. When Jill made rounds and found Mrs. Smith crying and upset, she recognized the patient's need for emotional support and sat down at her bedside to talk. Soon the physician came into the room complaining loudly that the test results were not on the chart and that he was in a hurry to leave the hospital. Jill explained that she would check into the status of the test results as soon as she was finished in that room and suggested, if the physician wanted immediate results, that he call the laboratory directly. He was outraged that Jill did not leave the patient's room immediately to find the results. Just then, the nursing supervisor arrived on the scene, asked for an explanation, apologized to the physician for the inconvenience, and left to track down the information.

Later that evening, the supervisor returned and, despite Jill's further explanation, criticized her for not responding sooner to the physician's request. Jill felt that she had been appropriately assertive with the physician but was disappointed that her efforts were not supported or rewarded. Why did Jill's supervisor not support her? One explanation may be that initially the supervisor did not have a clear picture of what had happened. The physician presented a very concrete situation: The laboratory results that he needed were unavailable. In this instance, Jill needed to be equally clear to the supervisor that she was involved in a therapeutic conversation with the patient and not social chit-chat. The assertive nurse assures that her boss has all the relevant facts.

A second possible explanation is that the supervisor did not realize she had a choice of responses or did not know how to follow through in another manner. In these instances, the assertive nurse can tactfully ask for support directly and even be specific about the action she wants. The nonassertive supervisor may respond positively to concrete suggestions and encouragement for assertive behavior on her part.

A third possible explanation for the supervisor's lack of support is that because she is not herself assertive or even aware of assertive concepts, she found it threatening to support an assertive subordinate. Consider that when a supervisor does muster the courage to support a nurse's assertive act, then usually the responsibility rests with the supervisor to defend the act to her boss. Indeed, the supervisor receives pressure from all sides, and to many individuals, this pressure is overwhelming. It is no wonder that nonassertive, insecure nurse managers are hesitant to send their staff to assertiveness programs or, if they do, say, "But don't use it on me!" It follows then that the supervisor needs to possess assertive skills also.

In addition to providing the opportunity to develop skills, nurse managers must reward assertive behavior. Some nurse managers are themselves assertive and do support and reward an assertive staff. At times, this may mean separating issues from behaviors. For instance, there may be occasions when the director of nursing disagrees with an assertive nurse on an issue and may not be able to grant a request but still can respect the nurse's right to express her opinion and acknowledge that she pursued the matter in a praiseworthy manner. When assertive behavior is supported in such a manner, it can transfer into instances where staff and management are working toward mutual goals.

Some nurse managers wisely resist pressure to stifle the so-called "rebel" or "maverick," especially if she behaves in a responsible manner. Actually, such nurses can be helpful to the nurse manager because when these nurses insist that their extremist views be considered, the more moderate position of the manager can be strengthened.

Peggy worked the evening shift at Hillside Hospital, a small general hospital located in a high-crime section of the city. There had been an increased incidence of theft, vandalism, and attempted rape in the hospital parking lot at night. Several well-lit parking spaces directly in front of the hospital were reserved for the medical staff. When Peggy and other evening nurses came to work, they were always directed by the parking attendant past the usually empty prime spaces to the poorly lit far end of the parking lot. Nursing management had tried several strategies to free at least half of the spaces for nurses but had been unsuccessful. The evening shift of nurses, with the support of nursing management, went through the proper channels within the hospital to gain access to the prime parking spaces, but they also failed.

In view of the unsafe conditions, Peggy felt strongly that the evening nurses had a right to the parking spaces and decided to pursue the matter further. So she wrote a letter about the unsafe situation to the editor of the local newspaper and the rape crisis center, and sent copies to the appropriate hospital authorities. Once the public was aware of the situation, the hospital administration and medical staff were pressured into sharing the prime parking spaces in the evening.

Because the hospital's public image had been challenged, the director of nursing was pressured to "fire the rebel." But this director reminded administration that if they had responded to the numerous original requests, the incident could have been avoided. Furthermore, while praising Peggy's persistence, she said that she needed more nurses like her in middle management and that she intended to promote Peggy when the next appropriate position became available.

While this is an extreme example, it does illustrate how sometimes an assertive staff can accomplish things that nursing management cannot because of its position in the organization. Sometimes these situations are perceived by staff to be a lack of support from nursing management, but, in reality, they reflect the nature of management and organizations. Because of factors unknown to the staff nurse, sometimes nursing management cannot support the staff's activities visibly. In these instances, it is important for the staff to realize that although they are not being supported actively, neither are they being blocked.

Nurse managers who sincerely want nurses to continue to function assertively are committed to creating a supportive work environment. Nurses and nursing will thrive in a positive work environment where open, frank discussions of issues are used as opportunities for growth and challenge. Nursing managers can participate in the thrust of assertiveness by emphasizing the positive when resolving problems and by offsetting the negativism that is so pervasive within the nursing profession. For instance, there needs to be less emphasis on assigning nurses negative labels such as "burned out" and less of the literature and educational programs devoted to such negative topics. While aiming to change these attitudes and behaviors and to improve the conditions that contribute to the formation of such nurses, nursing managers need to place these concerns in a more realistic perspective and acknowledge that, to a degree, such people and situations exist in all professions. Instead, we need to support nurses who pursue a positive, constructive approach to rectifying these problems once they have been identified.

An active educational approach wherein nursing students and current practitioners are purposefully taught assertive concepts and techniques must be ongoing and not regarded merely as a current fad or the latest "in vogue" trend. The continual development of assertive nurses and their benefit to patients and the nursing profession must be taken seriously. Given the current economic and social forces impacting on the nursing profession and the entire health care system, the need for assertive nurses will increase. Consequently, it is imperative for nurses at all levels to have the opportunity to develop assertive skills and to integrate support of assertive nurses into their daily work.

An assertive outlook can be used to accept the past, function more effectively in the present, and plan for a better tomorrow. Integrating assertive skills into planned change can help you to meet the challenges of the future, including the creation of new directions for nurses and nursing.

References

Benne, D., and M. Birnbaum. Principles of Changing. In *The Planning of Change,* edited by W. Bennis, K. Benne, and R. Chin, 2nd ed. New York: Holt, Rinehart & Winston, 1969.

Brooten, Dorothy, Laura Hayman, and Mary Naylor. *Leadership for Change: A Guide for the Frustrated Nurse.* Philadelphia: Lippincott, 1978.

Dalton, Gene, Paul Thompson, and Raymond Price. The Four Stages of Professional Careers: A New Look at Performance by Professionals. *Organizational Dynamics* 6 (1977):19–42.

Hertzberg, Frederick. *Work and the Nature of Man.* Columbus, Ohio: World Books, 1969.

Johnson, Bonnie. *Communication: The Process of Organizing.* Boston: Allyn & Bacon, 1977.

Kelly, Lucie Young. The Good New Nurse Network. *Nursing Outlook* 26 (1978):71.

Schaller, Lyle. *The Change Agent.* New York: Abington Press, 1972.

Spradley, Barbara Walton. Managing Change Creatively. *Journal of Nursing Administration* 10(5) (1980):32–37.

8
Assertively Influencing the Future

You can use your assertive skills in many ways to implement change for the advancement of the nursing profession; however, you are more likely to be successful if you concentrate on one or two areas of particular concern to you. The following three areas are discussed for your consideration: changing nursing's public image, influencing legislation, and influencing the health care system.

Changing Nursing's Public Image

Unfortunately, the public often associates professionally competent nurses exclusively with physicians or medical care. Although some nurses are quite satisfied to bask in this precarious prestige of medicine, nursing leaders urge nurses to define their practice more clearly as that of high-quality nursing rather than second-rate medicine. Possessing a positive self-image, the assertive nurse is comfortable and proud to be a nurse. Her attitude is not one of "I'm just a nurse" but rather "I'm a nurse . . . a competent health care professional." By using her skills to change inaccurate stereotypes, the assertive nurse enhances and promotes a more positive public image. This clarification can be achieved through existing opportunities such as participation in professional and service organizations, public relations groups, and interdisciplinary committees, and by writing for lay publications. New opportunities to define and promote nurses publicly are limited only by your imagination.

In addition to using assertive skills to promote a more accurate public image, the assertive nurse is also aware of how her individual appearance affects that image. Historically, nurses have been identified easily as the caregiver in the crisp white uniform and cap. As other health care providers adopted similar white uniforms and nurses stopped wearing the traditional cap, the identity of various workers has become obscure. While freedom from strict uniform codes is embraced as a welcome relief, the relaxed attitude of many nurses about their attire may be sending confusing or conflicting messages to others.

Ideally, people should be able to dress in whatever manner they choose and be treated as the individuals they are, not as what their attire represents. But in reality, most nurses work in male-dominated, sexist systems. If nurses want to be treated as professionals, their appearance and behavior need to convey professionalism. While one certainly can understand the interest of nurses in creating an individual look, nurses should learn from women in other professions and ask themselves the question, "What is my attire saying?" Many contemporary, aspiring businesswomen have become increasingly aware of the subtle role that appearance plays in how one is perceived (Henning and Jardim, 1976). Without returning to a matronly, neuter look or relying on repressive dress codes, an assertive nurse conveys a decisive, professional appearance; she is comfortable with her femininity but does not exploit it.

Thelma Schoor (1978) states that it is important for nurses to make a healthy, positive appearance in order to be viewed as competent by legislators and, consequently, to be consulted about health care issues. The same is true if nurses expect patients to listen and accept their health teaching. Schoor questions how competent or credible a nurse will be viewed by the public if she presents herself as an overweight chainsmoker who is inappropriately "squeezed into" a pantsuit or mini-skirted uniform.

Paying attention to your body and your appearance is a reflection of self-acceptance and self-confidence, both of which are related to assertiveness. Taking the time to evaluate your personal image conveys that your appearance did not just happen but rather that you make conscious decisions about your attire. While determining your own professional image can be another way of assuming responsibility for your life, it can also positively affect the collective public image of nursing.

Influencing Legislation

A second area affecting nursing that is significantly influenced by a collective approach is federal and state legislation, which allocates large sums of money for education and human services. As you become more self-confident and articulate in your personal and professional settings, a natural extension of using your assertive skills to promote professional advancement is to become involved with legislation and politics. Because most legislators are interested in listening to their constituents, communicating with them is an ideal opportunity for you to use your assertive skills outside your traditional setting. This can be done by visiting politicians' offices, communicating with them on nursing and health-related issues, or becoming involved in political campaigns. Your legislators' probable positive response will reinforce additional assertions on your part.

We echo other nursing writers in saying that most nurses are unaware of the potential political clout of individual nurses asserting their political influence. Individual political influence, keenly managed by a collaborative leadership, can create an extended power base for the profession. And because political issues can bridge diversity and initiate unified action, they can serve as a unifying factor. This unity has been demonstrated in many states where various groups of nurses have worked together to update Nurse Practice Acts. The political arena provides numerous opportunities for nurses to become more politically active, to tap into their potential collective power, and, consequently, to influence legislation assertively.

Influencing the Health Care System

While nurses can initiate change from within their segment of the health care system, they can further expand their areas of influence by pursuing positions at the top and on the periphery of these systems. As an example of the former, the nursing profession promotes a shift in the health care system from a focus on illness to that of wellness. In order for nurses to effect a change of this mag-

Developing the New Assertive Nurse

nitude, they must not only control the nursing care provided within the organization but must also significantly influence the future direction of service of the total organization. More directors of nursing must aspire to and become chief executive officers of health care systems.

Nurses also can influence the direction of health care from the periphery of the direct service organization by participation on various policy-making boards, including those of hospitals, local health departments, home health agencies, health planning associations, and other human service organizations. Investigate and actively choose what type of board appointment you prefer. To which board can you make the greatest contribution? Serving on a board can provide you with the opportunity to effect change, to extend your personal areas of influence, and to develop important liaisons.

In addition to working with health care providers, nurses should find creative ways to influence the large purchasers of health care, such as corporations. Corporations, which spend millions of dollars for health care, are an untapped resource that nursing has not yet addressed. As corporations become larger and spend more money on health care benefits for their employees, the services that they choose to fund will have a major impact on the availability and development of those services. Assertive nurses can play a major role in affecting the direction of health care by influencing corporate decisions about which employee benefits are purchased. Ideally, this influence is exerted at the board of directors' level. Nursing representation on such boards is certainly desirable and a goal toward which an assertive nurse may want to strive.

Other approaches that the assertive nurse may use to gain access to corporate decision makers include functioning as a consultant to industry and becoming recognized as an expert in the health care field. Nurses already employed by corporations and viewed as competent can influence these decision makers either by going through established channels or by pursuing informal networks.

Several avenues are open to nurses who are willing to assume an active role in this country's health care delivery system. Many knowledgeable and competent nurses have the ability to influence major health care decisions, but they need the support of others.

This support can be especially valuable in order to maintain assertive skills and to implement change.

Creating New Directions for Nurses and Nursing Through Assertiveness

Nursing today is part of a rapidly changing world that has undergone more change in the last 40 years than in the previous 2000. Some refer to the present time as an "historic movement" in which a multiplicity of major discoveries and events have converged to launch us into a new world order (Nesti, 1980). Consequently, not only is nursing facing the most rapid environmental changes in its history, but it is also challenged considerably from within the profession. It is experiencing turmoil, discomfort, and doubt. Within its constituency, practitioners are searching for equitable compensation, advancement, and fulfillment. Indeed, nurses are at a professional crossroads.

Nursing is confronted with trends that at first may appear to be insurmountable, but they must be regarded as invitations to set new directions assertively. We must expand our horizons and keep pace with our changing world. Unless we seek to review and update our original professional commitment with new dimensions, nursing's advancement will be in jeopardy. We must reexamine nursing's basic purpose and offer our vision and new insights, while keeping constant the profession's timeless commitment of providing service to others in a humanistic atmosphere of compassion and concern.

In our striving to effect change assertively and establish new directions for nursing, we must be careful not to discard meaningful aspects of our practice or abusively dismiss subgroups within our membership. Indeed, it would be advantageous for the profession if all of its diverse constituents were ambitious, full-time, career-oriented professionals with academic credentials in nursing and a genuine commitment to advancing themselves and the profession. While aspiring to such ideals, we need to recruit competent, enthusiastic, career-minded individuals into the profession and search for innovative ways to stimulate the development of these attributes in present nurses. However, in our aspirations, we must not demean those current practitioners whose choices or values differ from our own. Instead, we must be astute enough to recognize the potential benefits inherent in this time of turbulence and use our energies assertively in a positive way to develop and strengthen our membership for the future.

The assertive nurse (and ultimately, an assertive nursing profession) accepts the fact that nurses are a diverse professional group with varying value systems, credentials, and experiences—all of us with our own opinions and feelings about nursing and our places in the profession, and all of us believing that we have a right to function in a manner that is personally acceptable to us. This diversity gives nursing strength, balance, and flexibility, and can add to our status and contribution as a profession (Styles, 1981).

In our efforts to advance, we need to be realistic and realize that we cannot build a better profession for tomorrow unless we simultaneously meet the needs of the practitioners of today. We can accomplish this goal, at least in part, by helping ourselves and other nurses to grow and develop in self-satisfying and self-respectful ways. We must be aware that the climate in which tomorrow's nurse will be practicing will be influenced significantly by the nurses of today. In order for that climate to be conducive to the innovative ideas of the assertive new graduate, practicing nurses must also be assertive. An assertive practicing nurse will be open and receptive to the changes of others as well as actively initiating change herself. She will be eager to find "new directions" for the future.

In order to plan for the future effectively and deal with the external environmental forces impacting on the profession, it is necessary to establish a climate of trust within the profession. The advancement and progress that all of us yearn to see for nursing requires a commitment to such attributes as openness, honesty, and directness (in other words, assertiveness) in addition to patience, perseverence, and consistency. We must be consistent in what we say and do, especially in the way we initiate change. We must be consistent in the way we plan, implement our plans, and evaluate what we have done because of the importance of establishing trust among ourselves. A cohesive, progressive profession is comprised of competent, satisfied individuals who feel good about themselves. Developing an assertive attitude and acting in an assertive manner is one way of attaining this goal.

The future of nursing and the provision of quality patient care are closely intertwined. Assertive nurses will greatly enhance both. While the development of assertive techniques centers primarily on the self, a truly assertive attitude exemplified in an assertive life-style goes far beyond the self. Centering on the self simply provides a basis for a healthier external focus outside the self. As a result of the self-nourishment that occurs through internalizing the concepts of assertiveness, the nurse can reach out and give to patients in a more effective way. The assertive nurse realizes that she has a responsibility to develop and improve herself so that she can serve her patients and her profession better. In turn, she realizes that she also has a right to be fulfilled, recognized, rewarded, and valued for her efforts.

As the integration of assertive behavior permeates the nursing profession and we join together, a new image of nursing will emerge. The internal strife that exists within and between individuals and subgroups will be superseded by a shared vision and a common purpose. We must all participate in the search for a new and better profession by sharing our abilities in order to develop the potential and creativity of our nursing colleagues. Working to coordinate our diverse interests is central to the strategic planning so essential for our future. By renewing and reinforcing our efforts to collaborate, we will meet the major challenges that lie ahead. We will view nursing as "one profession [united] under one fundamental belief about who we are and what we are destined to achieve" (Styles, 1981, p. 10).

While persisting toward our goal of forming new directions for nursing, we must purposefully remind ourselves of the progress already made. We must also dedicate ourselves to the proposition that "nursing is a vital force for social progress . . . which provides a distinct, vital perspective and service offered by no other health profession" (Styles, 1981, p. 10). We have to view ourselves and our profession as worthy, valuable contributors to the health care system. Recognizing and utilizing this uniqueness to attain advancement for nurses and nursing is assertiveness in action.

Our goal for the emergence of a "new" nursing profession

cannot be achieved by individuals who are afraid to be assertive; afraid to take risks and to pay the price; afraid to feel the exertion, to stretch, to move, to change, or to accept the discomfort that is involved in growth and change. In breaching the gap between what is acceptable today and imaginable tomorrow:

- We invite you to make informed choices, to be a risk taker, and to be persistent in your assertive attempts to bring about change.

- We invite you to refuse to be victimized by apathy and discouragement, to develop self-control, and to maintain a positive assertive attitude directed toward progress and advancement.

- We invite you to put things in perspective by keeping in touch with your own humanness, with the aspects of caring and service to others as you carry out your life's work, and to allow room for happiness, joy, and laughter in the serious business of reshaping nursing.

- We invite you to call forth your creativity to make your assertive contribution in meeting nursing's changing needs and designing its new directions.

- And, above all, we invite you to be assertive in reaffirming your importance and value to nursing and to society . . . the value that you have been, that you are, and that you are becoming.

References

Henning, Margaret, and Ann Jardim. *The Managerial Woman.* Englewood Cliffs, N.J.: Doubleday, 1976.

Nesti, Donald. Inaugural Address. Duquesne University, Pittsburgh, Pennsylvania, Fall 1980.

Schoor, Thelma M. As Others See Us. *American Journal of Nursing* (September 1978):1477.

Styles, Margretta. Unity and Diversity: Partners in the 80s. *Pennsylvania Nurse* (January 1981):10.

Index

Acceptance of others, 102–106
Accountability
 and individual rights, 96–97
 and responsibility, 142–146
Aggressive behavior, 8–11
Aggressive nonverbal communication, 126
Alternatives, assessing, 62–69
Anger
 blocking assertiveness, 155–156
 dealing assertively with another person's, 153–155
 direct expressions of, 161–164
 handling your own, 157–164
 indirect expressions of, 159–161
 as a motivator, 157–164
 recognizing displaced, 156–157
 and refusals, 151–152
 resolution of, 165–166
 self-control and, 264–265
Anticipating, art of, 178–180
Anxiety and assertiveness, 173–176
Assertive action and attentive listening, 116–117
Assertive Checklist, 192, 213–217
Assertiveness
 and acceptance of others, 102–106
 advantages of, 32–36
 versus aggressive behavior, 8–11
 anger and, 153–166
 anxiety and, 173–176
 Bill of Assertive Rights, 77–84
 as a choice, 7–8, 28–29, 32–33, 36–73, 106–109
 communication and, see Communication
 criticism and, 166–170
 cyclic effect of successful, 177–178
 decision making and, 36–73
 definition of, 7–8
 disadvantages of, 32–36
 inhibitors of, overcoming, 137–176
 irrational beliefs and, 137–141, 148–152
 and nonverbal communication, 123–127
 versus passive behavior, 8–11
 planning and, 180–184
 promoters of, 177–199
 put-downs and, 170–173
 reasons to learn, 5–7
 refusals and, 140–153
 skill-building techniques, 185–194
 using skills to implement change, 201–232
Assertive nonverbal communication, 127
Assertive response/approach, components of, 25–28, 190–191
Assertive techniques, 25–28
Assertive verbal communication, 118–123
Assessment for change, 206, 209–212

Beliefs
 irrational, 137–141, 148–152
 rational, 138–141, 148–152
 and values, 40–41